Natural Remedies For

Dog Diseases

Mark Gilberd
Homoeopath. Medical Herbalist and Iridologist

Index

Materia Medica

Staphysagria, Symphytum, Tarantula Cuba, Urtica Urens.

The Safest Essential Oils For Animal Use

How Oils Work

Oils For Dogs

How Oils Work

The Golden Rules

Shampoo Formula

Oil Blends _ Formulas

Oils For Horses

The Essentials Below Are Fairly Safe For Animal Use

Introduction
Welcome To The Animal Natural Remedy Series

These books are a effort to preserve the documentation of Natural Remedies used in the treatment of animals. In the past 100 years most of these treatments have been lost, especially in the treatment of cattle one of our most ancient of farm animals. Other reasons for writing these books is that I hate vet bills and people having to kill their farm animals or pets for economic reasons which I myself have been forced to do in the past on a Goat farm. Originally these books were put together as a field reference for myself for there is nothing worse than being in a paddock with a sick animal with the farmer, his hands on his hips waiting for you to perform and fix his animal.

Now the books have evolved and have had about 15 years of additions and are offered to you to teach you a new way of thinking. The books have evolved more by my different trainings. As a farmer I learnt to supplement the animals with the deficiencies of the soil so the books always start with the vitamins and minerals and their deficiency symptoms. As a Iridologist I tend to think and work with Body Systems such as The Nervous System or The Digestive System and concentrate on building them up with Nutrition and Herbs. As a Medical Herbalist I am trained to think holistically and design formulas that cover the whole being along with making the formulas easily absorbed. My Homoeopathic training teaches me to pay attention to the mind symptoms and to pay attention to what is really there not what I think is there and to treat and relieve the symptoms of the individual. Homoeopathy also shows how disease taints can be inherited and what to look for and how to treat them but best of all it gives me a special weapon to use when disaster strikes in the form of epidemics, these are called Disease Nosodes which are a preparation made from the disease product so you have a tool to help prevent the spread of disease. The books are set out in such a way as to teach you the correct use of Herbs eg thinking in body systems such as the Respiratory System or the Nervous System and in using herbs by their Medical Actions rather then that herb worked well last time. At the end of each system for example The Nervous System we have a section that gives you the common Actions used and needed for that section. Keeping with our example The Nervous System some of our Actions would be Anti-spasmodic, Sedative and Nervine Stimulants. After the explanation of the Action you have a list of herbs that are known to be strong in that action, this gives you more of a selection of herbs then what is mentioned in the text. Next we move on to the Homoeopathic Remedies for the condition which have the details to allow you to select a reasonably similar remedy. Homeopathy sits on a three legged stool. What this means is that if a remedy has at least three symptoms in the same strength as the symptoms you are trying to match then that remedy is a potential cure for your patient or if not cure it will offer the condition relief. The more symptoms you can match to the remedy the better the remedy will work for the rule is likes cure likes not vaguely similar cures. Homoeopathy (homo means same pathy means disease) is a good form of treatment for animals who usually respond to it fairly well and also it is very cheap to use and very easy to medicate unlike the herbs. A lot of effort has been put into the symptom details of the disease as it is very hard trying to diagnose when the animal can't answer your questions, so here you have to be very observant.

If used correctly this book makes you think and act more like a Professional Herbalist and broadens your view on what you are doing. With the Homoeopathics I have only really given you the leading remedies to put you on the right track, it would be worthwhile to invest in a good Materia Medica (Homoeopathic Remedy Reference) such as Boericke's which is one of the best for the Layman.

Main Reference Sources

The original base of the herbs I use were sourced from Juliette de Baïracli Levy's old Herbals, as hers are about the only Animal Herb References that have not been lost in time and they give you a lot of the old ancient herbs that have been used throughout most of history. To these I have added a lot of the more modern Herbs especially those that I use in my own work such as Astragalus and those that will soon be added after using for the first time on animals because there are just no substitutes. A good and recent example is Brahmi which I used in a cat recovering from a stroke because of my previous success in humans with this herb as it is supposed to rewire the brain around the damaged area and in its 3000 years of constant use someone must of used it on an Animal before. There are new herbs coming mainly from the Philippines, Indonesia, India and China but they are still being tried and tested and the average person wouldn't be able to get hold of them but the future looks far brighter than what it was 15 years ago when I started slowly putting this all together. We owe a lot to Juliette de Baïracli Levy for without her all these valuable herbs and how they were used would be lost. She has created a strong foundation that we can now build on.

Juliette de Baïracli Levy (11 November 1912 – 28 May 2009) was an English herbalist and author noted for her pioneering work in holistic veterinary medicine. Born to a wealthy Jewish family (her father was Turkish, her mother Egyptian) and raised in England with chauffeurs, maids, cooks, and gardeners. She knew as a child that she wanted to be a veterinarian. After studying veterinary medicine at the Universities of Manchester and Liverpool for two years she left England to study herbal medicine in Europe, Turkey, North Africa, Israel and Greece, living with gypsies, farmers and livestock breeders and recording their knowledge, especially the

Gypsies. "I realized that if I wanted to learn the traditional ways of healing and caring for animals, I had to be where people still lived close to the land and close to their flocks," she says. "From Berbers, Bedouins, nomads, peasants, and gypsies in England, Israel, Greece, Turkey, Mexico, and Austria, I learned herbal knowledge and the simple laws of health and happiness. I never tired of traveling with my Afghan Hounds, always living with and learning from those around me." After living for some time on the Greek island Kythira she then resided in an old age home in Burgdorf, Switzerland leaving the world a better place.

For Homoeopathy my main hero is George Macleod not only for the success had based on his work but in my opinion he is a Homoeopathic Master up there with the greats and I admire his work in the use of Homoeopathic Disease Nosodes. All the high potencies mentioned are his work along with most of the Nosodes for as any trained Homoeopath knows and has had beaten into them during training you don't change the work of the masters. Unfortunately in our fast paced world not many people have time for Homoeopathy but I will say this, in the next Global Pandemic I and my family will be safe because I will make the Disease Nosode of it for I was trained by the Homoeopathic Masters.

George MacLeod (McLeod) (1912 – 1995) MRCVS DVSM Veterinary FF. Hom was a homeopathic vet, President of The British Association of Homeopathic Vets, Veterinary Consultant to The Homeopathic

Development Foundation. George MacLeod was a graduate of Glasgow University and was one of the world's foremost authorities on Homeopathic treatment of animals. He was one of the few veterinary surgeons to use Homeopathic medicines wholly and exclusively. He was responsible for keeping Homeopathy available for animals in the UK, almost single-handedly, for the middle part of the 20th Century.

Other animal Homoeopaths sourced are Christopher Day, Edward Ruddock, and John Rush

Animal Natural Remedy Books

Natural Remedies For Cat Health
Natural Remedies For Dog Health
Natural Remedies For Goat Health
Natural Remedies For Sheep Health
Natural Remedies For Pig Health
Natural Remedies For Cow Health
Natural Remedies For Horse Health
Natural Remedies For Poultry Health

Mark Gilberd, Homoeopath, Iridologist, Medical Herbalist
Accredited With The Australian Traditional Medicine Society

Temperature, Heart Rate and Pulse

Temperature

The normal temperature for a dog ranges between 37.8 C (100F) and 39.2C (102.%).

A elevated temperature is often a sign of infection, pain or stress, or just excitement.

A temperature below normal usually indicates a debilitating disease or disorder.

How to take the Temperature.

1. Use a glass thermometer.

2. Shake the mercury down and smear the end with Vaseline.

3. Insert the thermometer into the dogs anus to about 5cm or 2 inches.

4. Withdraw the thermometer after about one or two minutes and check the reading.

Heart Rate and Pulse

The normal pulse and heart rate of a dog varies according to bread, age, weight etc. Normal ranges are from 80 to 100 beats per minute. To obtain correct readings the dog must be calm and relaxed.

Checking the Pulse

The best place to check your dog's pulse rate is the femoral artery, which runs along the thigh bone on the inside of the hind leg, about half way between the hip and the knee. You will feel a distinct groove between the muscles there. Place your fingers into this groove using gentle pressure and feel for the pulse. Count the number of beats for 15 seconds and multiply by four to get the number of beats per minute. The pulse should feel strong and fall within the normal range. If the pulse is rapid, weak or erratic you may have problems.

Checking the Heartbeat

The heartbeat is best located behind the left elbow and between the 3rd and 6th rib. The beat can also be observed as a regular slight movement in the same area.

De-Sexing Your Animals

In Australia over 300,000 unwanted, homeless and abandoned cats and dogs are put down each year so why do we want to bring more in the world when we can't even look after what is here already. I believe it is best to wait till the animal is mature and its organs are fully developed before de-sexing. De-sexing is best done just after puberty for females maybe 6 to 8 months and for males you should wait a little while longer as they are more slow to mature then females maybe about 9 to 12 months.

Animals that are not De-sexed may have mating urges that can lead to behavior that is considered undesirable by some humans such as running away, fighting other animals of the same sex and getting injured, territorial marking, yowling and climbing walls, females being pursued by male animals, hyperactivity or aggression.

De-sexing does not take away the animals zest for life or make them lazy, it makes animals less prone to prostate cancer and reproductive diseases and on average they live longer.

Vaccinations

I am very unsure about vaccinations and after reading of the side effects in humans from the manuals that Doctors use to vaccinate I find the whole idea fairly disturbing and I have never yet seen a document proving beyond a doubt that vaccinations truly work and there is just so much disinformation out there I don't think the truth will ever be known until it is possibly to late. It seems strange that Allopathic Medicine which usually always insists that they have to have proof, that there has to be double blind studies etc and as yet we have never really seen the proof.

I know that animals suffer a lot of complications from the vaccines that they are given but when vaccinations make up about a big part of your vets income and make the drug companies millions we will no doubt have to put up with lots more disinformation for many years to come.

I would be very interested in the results of a survey of how many vets vaccinate their own animals. A lot of you may be forced to vaccinate your pet if you ever put them in a veterinary hospital or ever need to board your cat or dog in a boarding kennel. The question to ask here if this happens to you is why should I vaccinate my animal when all of yours are already vaccinated or don't your vaccines work?. I can see the argument they will use against this but let's use their claims against them, surely your animals should be safe because they have been vaccinated and obviously they can't give the disease to my pet because they have been vaccinated and can't get the disease.

If You Must Vaccinate

1. Wait at least till the animal is 3 months old so the immune system has had a chance to mature.
2. Never vaccinate a animal with symptoms of acute or chronic health problems, or at the time of surgery or any other physical or emotional stress.
3. Try to vaccinate for one disease at a time allowing time for recovery and only used killed vaccines not live modified virus vaccines.
4. Does a animal in good health on a good diet instead of the usual junk food diet really need boosters ?, and if you decide yes then why not do it every two to three years especially if your pet is in the middle years.

Bad Effects of Vaccination

Signs of a negative vaccine effect are - erratic behavior problems soon after shots, small warts, cancer, kidney failure, tumors, bloat of the stomach, skin problems, some say that 90% of skin problems are related to toxic vaccination and some animals have actually contracted the disease they were vaccinated for especially in Feline Leukemia and Parvo.

Homoeopathic Treatment

If you suspect the cats or dogs illness is related to

vaccinations directly after the vaccinations or three months down the track you can reduce the toxic side effects by using

Thuja 30C - as soon as possible dose nightly for seven nights then dose with Sulphur 30C weekly for seven more doses.

Herbal Treatment

A natural antidote which acts as a body cleanser and as a detoxifier for vaccinosis reaction whether they are tumors or skin problems are a combination of Sweet Violets and Red Clover.

Diet And Nutrition

Our Supermarket Pet food

The supermarket and Pet Food manufactures do not provide safe food for our pets even though the adds tell us that they do but the simple fact is just read the can where it says Not Fit For Human Consumption . If you can't eat it why expect your pet to. Now let's have a look where all this food comes from. 40% of the food comes from the rubbish parts of the slaughter trade being mainly feet, organs, blood, hides, hooves, beaks etc, (I know as I used to drive the tilt forklift with the buckets of offal which I used to tilt over the freezer while another person sorted by putting the heart in one section, liver in another etc) and we won't mention the animals that are diseased and cancerous that failed to meet the grade for human consumption.

The remaining percentage of our supermarket pet

foods consist of vegetable fibre, grain and chemicals. Vegetable fibre is made up of corn husks, peanut hulls, ground up corn and what a nutrition-less waste it is. In many cases it is grain or soy meal which has been condemned from human consumption because of mold, debris, odors or bacterial contamination.

Next come the chemicals, but before we get to that lets have a look at the chemicals which are feed and medicated to the beef and poultry and other farm animal so as to bring them to slaughter earlier and allow them to live in crowded conditions, these mainly are hormones, steroids and antibiotics. Obviously these chemicals would be concentrated in some organs especially the liver which has the job of getting rid of them so they would be bound to pass on to all who eat them. Now add to these chemicals all the ones that are now added to preserve the product with the worst being Ethoxyquin (Find out about this one yourself especially who invented it and for what purpose as I don't want to be run over by a pet food truck). Now after this comes the artificial colorings, sugar (diabetes) and salt (blood pressure, kidney problems) which prevent the fat in the food from going rancid. Sugar can comprise as much as 25% of the semi moist dog food packets and dog biscuits. Sugar and salt can become addictive, resulting in diabetes, arthritis, cataracts, allergies, overweight, tooth decay and nervousness. In other words we have given them all our human problems which we get from eating processed foods. So next time you are in the supermarket buying pet food read the labels very carefully and ask lots of questions.

Let's have a look now what a proper diet should be.

What The Diet Should Be

Dogs and cats are both carnivores which are flesh eaters and as such require a diet of flesh derived protein, raw meat is the central ingredient in a optimal diet. This meat for our pets should be of human consumption quality, fed raw because cooking destroys the vitamins, minerals and enzymes needed for digestion. Cooked and canned food is dead food for our pets and causes mucous to form in the animals intestines, mucous being the main food for worms and parasites.

A good diet would be of about 75% raw meat eg beef, poultry, fish etc and about 25% vegetables. The Vegetables could include very finely chopped carrots, broccoli, sprouts, parsley, asparagus, garlic, sweet potatoes, squash, cauliflower, turnips etc.

The best type of food you can feed your cat or dog is the one you make yourself. It is the most natural, the most nutritionally balanced; the most easily digested and of much higher quality then canned or dry pet food.

Homemade pet food is not only free of harmful additives but has the added benefit of being able to include herbs. Two good ones that should be used frequently are garlic which is a natural anti biotic which has a high sulphur content which acts as a natural flea repellent and the other herb is parsley that acts on the urinary system keeping it free from problems. A good diet produces a good and healthy digestive system which makes it very hard for worms and parasites to survive and also eliminates constipation. For those who feel that they do not have the time to prepare homemade food you will be happy to know that you can prepare it all at once and freeze maybe a week's worth at a time. Really it does not cost much more than what you spend on pet food anyway and just imagine how much money you will save yourself in future vet bills.

Let's take a look now at the digestive systems of cats and dogs and see why this diet is suitable.

Cats and dogs do not chew their food for their teeth are for ripping and tearing and they swallow their food in chunks. Their digestive systems are much more acidic then ours and the small intestines are much shorter so meat goes through very quickly. Raw vegetables must be processed into very fine tiny pieces in order for the carnivore to digest them properly and be able to utilize them. In nature carnivores would get pre-digested vegetation while eating the stomach of a herbivore that they had killed. In preparing foods for our animals we do not have the option of feeding pre-digested vegetables so we must do what we can to provide raw ground vegetables which are as close to what Mother Nature would do as possible.

The Dog Diet - Natural and Home Prepared

50% Raw Meat - chopped or diced mutton, goat, roo, fish or organic chicken.. Minced meat destroys B vitamins, cooked meat destroys digestive enzymes making proper digestion very difficult. Once a month feed organ meat eg raw liver is highly nutritious. Throughout the week natural cottage cheese, goats milk, cooked eggs or if raw egg yolk only can be feed without any problems.

40% Vegies - (anything yellow or green). Make sure that they are finely grated or diced for easy digestion. If cooked best to use pumpkin well mashed if uncooked pulp from a juicer or well mulched carrot and or zucchini.

No - onions, potatoes, peas, cabbage , citrus fruits or pork.

10% Herbs - Add daily about 1 tablespoon of finely chopped parsley (cleanses kidneys of toxins) and garlic finely chopped or minced into meals, quarter clove for pets under 5kg, 1 clove for 10 to 30kg and 2 cloves for 40kg.

Note - Try to vary the foods so the dog does not become bored with the diet.

Bones - must be raw, best are lamb shank bones for medium to large dogs. Avoid marrow bones as they are too hard and wear the teeth down. Cooked bones of any sort or sun bleached bones may splinter and perforate the stomach. On a all-natural diet it is very important to add supplements to obtain a balanced diet of vitamins, minerals and fatty acids and if you add barley grass you will also be adding the essential amino acids as well.

Supplements For The Dog.

Vitamin and Mineral Powder Supplement

Mix the powder supplements together and store in an air tight container
1 cup of Bonemeal or Dolomite Powder
1/3 Cup of Kelp Powder
Half a Cup of Lecithin Grains

Essential Fatty Acids Oil Supplement

1 and a quarter Cup of cold pressed Safflower Oil (EFAs)
Half a Cup of Flaxseed Oil (omega 3,6,9 and Vit E)
Quarter of a Cup of Cod Liver Oil (Vit A and D)
All of these natural vitamin and mineral supplements can be found at good health stores.

Daily Dosage By Dogs Weight

2 to 8kg - teaspoon of powder and 1 teaspoon of oil mix

8 to 14 - teaspoon of powder and 2 teaspoons of oil mix

15 to 24.- teaspoon and a half of powder and half a tablespoon of oil mix.

25 to 36 - 2 teaspoons of powder and 1 tablespoon of oil mix.

Plus add to each evening meal Ester C Powder (vitamin C)

1/8 of a teaspoon for a small dog

1/4 of a teaspoon for medium dog

1/2 of a teaspoon for large dog

Apple Cider Vinegar aids digestion and is a general health tonic; 2 teaspoons full can be put in the water or food.

B - Complex 50 to 70mg can be given to animals that are stressed, nervous or are recovering from surgery or injury. Also give for behavior disorder - chewing, hyperactivity etc., crush tablet and add to meals. Brewer's yeast is a good source of the B vitamins

Barley Green Powder - can be added to meals for extra nutrition especially when the pet is sick or unwell. Add 3 teaspoons to meals.

Evening Primrose Oil - is vital to the immune system and contains GLA, Vit E and omega 6 and 9. Good for pets suffering from arthritis, skin disease, hormone problems and bone degenerative diseases. Add 1 teaspoon to meals.

Nutritional Requirements For Adult Dogs

Protein

Source - Meat, fish, milk, eggs.

Function - Builds bones and repairs tissue. Maintains growth

Deficiency - Slow growth, weak or deformed bones.

Excess - Obesity, brittle bones.

Fat

Source – Animal and vegetable fats and oils.

Function - Provides energy and healthy skin, aids metabolic processes.

Deficiency - Dull coat, delayed healing of wounds.

Excess - Obesity, liver disease.

Carbohydrate

Source - Cereals, rice, pasta, potatoes.

Function - Provides energy and is a source of bulk in the diet.

Deficiency - Possible fertility and whelping problems.

Excess – Obesity

Minerals And Vitamins

Calcium

Function - Assists in the contraction of muscles. Required for blood clotting. Assists in the production of hormones and enzymes. Works with phosphorus and Vitamin D to produce bone, bone is 35 percent calcium.

Sources – Milk, cheese, bones and milk.

Herb Sources - Alfalfa, Blue Cohosh, Chamomile, Cleavers, Coltsfoot, Cayenne, Comfrey, Dandelion, Kelp, Mistletoe, Meadowsweet, Nettles, Parsley, Plantain, Raspberry, Rose Hips, Shepherds Purse, Yarrow, Yellow Dock.

Deficiencies - Rickets in young, Developmental Orthopaedic Disease, Azoturia, Poor muscle function, Impaired blood clotting, Joint problems and bone weakness.

Phosphorous

Function - Works with calcium for bone growth. Assists in energy metabolism. Makes up 15 percent of bone. Too much phosphorous will reduce the absorption of calcium during digestion.

Sources – Milk, bones and meat.

Herb Sources - Alfalfa, Anise, Asparagus, Blue Cohosh, Caraway, Cayenne, Chickweed, Calamus, Dandelion, Dill, Fenugreek, Garlic, Golden Rod, Kelp, Licorice, Linseed, Marigold, Meadowsweet, Parsley,

Raspberry, Rose Hips, Sunflower, Yellow Dock.

Deficiencies - Overfeeding of phosphorous can lead to lameness, fragile bones, enlargement of the jaw bone, hyperparathyroidism

Magnesium

Function - Required for hemoglobin formation in the blood. Assists in bone formation. Assists in enzyme functions of the body.

Sources – Bones, fish , dark green vegetables.

Herb Sources - Alfalfa, Blue Cohosh, Broom, Carrot leaves, Cayenne, Dandelion, Hops, Marshmallow, Meadowsweet, Mistletoe, Mullein, Peppermint, Raspberry, Slippery Elm.

Deficiencies - Nervousness and excitability. Increased respiratory rates. Muscle tremors. Aggressiveness and ill temper.

Sulphur

Function – Contained in amino acids methionine and cystine. Assists in enzyme and hormone production.

Sources – Meat and eggs.

Herb Sources - Alfalfa, Burdock, Broom, Calamus, Coltsfoot, Cayenne, Daisy, Eyebright, Fennel, Garlic, Kelp, Marigold, Meadowsweet, Mullein, Nettle, Parsley, Plantain, Raspberry, Sage, Shepherds purse, Thyme, Yarrow.

Deficiencies – Poor growth and coat.

Sodium Chloride

Function - Maintains the balance of fluids in the cells. Assists in muscle contractions. Removes waste products from the cells. Required in the production of bile. Maintains the health of the nervous system.

Sources - Salt and salt licks and cereals.

Deficiencies - Dehydration, Poor Growth, hair loss, muscle cramps. Over feeding of salt can result in high blood pressure.

Potassium

Function - Works with sodium to assist in correct nerve function and muscular contractions. Assists in maintaining the correct fluid balance in the body.

Herb Sources - Alfalfa, Blue Cohosh, Borage, Carrot leaves, Chamomile, Coltsfoot, Comfrey, Couch Grass, Centaury, Dandelion, Elder, Eyebright, Fennel, Kelp, Ladies Mantle, Mistletoe, Meadowsweet, Mullein, Nettles, Parsley, Peppermint, Plantain, Raspberry, Shepherds Purse, Skullcap, Wormwood, Yarrow.

Source – Milk and meat.

Deficiencies - Weight loss, Diarrhea, Muscle weakness and heart problems

Zinc

Function - Assists in the metabolism of nutrients. Required for the immune system to function correctly. Needed for healthy skin, hair and nails.. Assists in blood formation.

Sources - Yeast, Bran, Cereal Germ and Zinc Sulphate.

Herb Sources - Kelp and Marshmallow.

Deficiencies - Can lead to dry flaky skin, hair loss and poor growth loss.

Copper

Function - Essential in the formation of hemoglobin, cartilage and bone. Required for the correct utilization of iron in the body.

Sources – Meat and bones.

Herb Sources - Burdock, Chickweed, Chicory, Dandelion, Fennel, Garlic, Horseradish, Kelp, Parsley, Yarrow.

Deficiencies - Brittle weak bones, anemia, faded dull coat, in foals copper deficiency is associated with osteochondritis.

Manganese

Function - Required for the utilization of fats and carbohydrates. Essential for the formation of cartilage, assists in the formation of bones and enzymes.

Sources – Cereals and nuts.

Herb Sources - Kelp.

Deficiencies – Poor growth and fertility.

Iron

Function - Essential for the formation of hemoglobin and red blood cells.

Sources – Meat and vegetables.

Herb Sources - Alfalfa, Asparagus, Bilberry, Burdock, Blue Cohosh, Cayenne, Chicory, Comfrey, Dandelion, Gentian, Hawthorn, Hops, Mullein, Nettles, Parsley, Raspberry, Skullcap, Vervain, Yellow Dock.

Deficiencies - Anemia, Poor Performance, Poor growth..

Fluorine

Function - Essential for the formation of healthy teeth and bones, helps prevent tooth decay. Combines with calcium in the body and gives strength to the bones.

Sources - Water and Limestone based supplements.

Herb Sources - Alfalfa, Beet leaves, Garlic, Water Cress.

Deficiencies - Deficiencies are rare but overdosing can occur. Signs of overdosing are discolored, mottled teeth, poor condition and rough coat and lameness in the joints.

Iodine

Function - Needed for correct functioning of the thyroid gland. Required for reproductive cycle to function correctly.

Sources – Kelp and fish.

Herb Sources - Asparagus, Cleavers, Garlic, Kelp, Speedwell, Sarsaparilla.

Deficiencies - Abnormal oestrous cycle and slow metabolism. Overdosing can lead to enlarged thyroid glands.

Selenium

Function - Works with Vitamin E. Essential part of antioxidant enzymes which help which help to remove toxins from the system. A component of the amino acids Methionine and Cystine. Assists in maintaining a healthy immune system.

Sources – Fish meal meat and cereals.

Deficiencies – Cause muscle problems. Over supplementing can cause poisoning.

Vitamins

Vitamin A (retinol)

Function - Needed for hormone synthesis, bone growth, and used in most of the mucous membranes of the body.

Sources - Carrots, Carotene in green leafy plants ,

milk, and Cod Liver Oil.

Herb Sources - Alfalfa, Burdock, Cayenne, Comfrey, Dandelion, Kelp, Marshmallow, Papaya, Parsley, Raspberry, Red Clover, Watercress, Yellow Dock.

Deficiencies - Night blindness, Excessive tears, Rough coat, Lack of appetite, Infections of the reproductive tract, Poor growth and weak bones and tendons.

B1 Thiamine

Function - Assists in metabolizing carbohydrates. Maintains a healthy nervous system. Assists in energy metabolism. Has been found to have a calming effect. Can assist in the performance and stamina.. This vitamin is made by microflora in the intestines.

Sources – Peas, beans, organ meat, whole grains and Brewer's Yeast.

Herb Sources - Alfalfa, Burdock, Cayenne, Comfrey, Dandelion, Kelp, Marshmallow, Papaya, Parsley, Raspberry, Red Clover, Watercress, Yellow Dock.

Deficiencies - Weight loss, Muscular in coordination and missed heart beats. Deficiencies are fairly rare due to this vitamin being made in the intestines.

B2 Riboflavin

Function - Maintains a healthy nervous system.

Assists in energy metabolism. This vitamin is also made in the intestines.

Sources – Cheese, meat and milk.

Herb Sources - Alfalfa, Burdock, Fenugreek, Kelp, Parsley, Watercress.

Deficiencies - Rough coat and dry skin, Conjunctivitis, Excessive tearing and may be connected with moon blindness. Deficiencies are fairly rare.

B3 Niacin

Function - Helps in the metabolism of nutrients and also with hormone and lipid syntheses. This vitamin is also made in the intestines.

Sources – Meat, cereals and legumes.

Herb Sources - Alfalfa, Burdock, Fenugreek, Kelp, Parsley, Sage.

Deficiencies – Mouth ulcers Over dosing may cause dilation of blood vessels, sickness and itching of skin.

B5 Pantothenic Acid

Function - Assists in energy metabolism and the formation of anti-bodies.

Sources - Cereals and Peas.

Deficiencies - Deficiency is rare as this vitamin is made in the intestines.

B6 Pyridoxine

Function - Assists in energy metabolism. Maintains health of the nervous system. Assists in the formation of hemoglobin in the blood. Maintains the health of the immune system.. This vitamin is made in the bowel.

Sources – Meat, vegetables, cereals and eggs.

Herb Sources - Alfalfa, Chlorophyll.

Deficiencies - Anorexia, anemia, weight loss and convulsions.

B12 Cyanocobalamin

Function - Assists in the production of red blood cells. Assists in energy metabolism. Can assist in putting on condition and correcting anemia. This vitamin is made in the bowel.

Sources – Meat, eggs and milk

Herb Sources - Alfalfa, Chlorophyll, Dong Quai, Kelp.

Deficiencies - None recorded.

Biotin

Function - Assists in the metabolism of energy. Can assist in the improvement of poor quality hooves in some horses. Maintains sebaceous glands in the skin. Maintains bone marrow.

Sources – Meat and vegetables.

Deficiencies – Scaly skin.

Choline

Function - Assists in the transport of fats stored in the liver to other areas of the body for use as energy. Maintains a healthy nervous system.

Sources - Natural Fats, eggs, liver, cereals peas and beans.

Deficiencies - Can lead to poor growth and increased storage of fats in the liver.

Folic Acid

Function - Assists cell metabolism. Required for red blood cell formation. Assists in general metabolism.

Sources - Green leafy forage

Deficiencies - None recorded in horses

Vitamin C (ascorbic acid)

Function - Essential for the formation of collagen tissue which is vital in tendons and cartilage. Essential for the utilization of essential amino acids lysine and proline.

Sources – Fruit, vegetables and can be supplemented in disease.

Herb Sources - Alfalfa, Burdock, Catnip, Cayenne, Chickweed, Dandelion, Hawthorn, Garlic, Horseradish, Kelp, Parsley, Plantain, Papaya, Raspberry, Rosehips, Shepherds Purse, Yellow Dock.

Deficiencies - None recorded. Supplementation has

been given in periods of stress and growth.

Vitamin D

Function - Essential for the absorption of calcium and for growth maintenance and repair of bones and teeth.

Sources – Milk, cheese, eggs, cod liver oil and through the skin after contact with sunlight.

Herb Sources - Alfalfa, Chlorophyll, Don Quai, Kelp.

Deficiencies - Reduced growth, rickets, weak bones and increased bone problems.

Vitamin E

Function - Helps with the immune system and is a powerful antioxidant. Helps stabilize cell membranes and acts on the reproductive system.

Sources – Cheese, green vegetables, cereals and Alfalfa.

Herb Sources - Alfalfa, Dandelion, Dong Quai, Kelp, Raspberry, Rose Hips, Water Cress.

Deficiencies - Anemia, Swelling of joints, muscular in coordination and weakness, reduced stamina.

Vitamin K

Function - Helps in the clotting of blood and in calcium assimilation.

Sources – Meat, green vegetables, liver.

Herb Sources - Alfalfa, Chlorophyll, Plantain, Shepherds Purse.

Deficiencies - Bleeding and longer blood clotting time.

Notes

Diseases Of the Respiratory System

Dogs generally have a robust and healthy respiratory system but when trouble does appear pay immediate attention to it for the condition can get worse very quickly. Learn to recognize yours dogs normal breathing and behavior so you will notice when something is wrong. Some pedigree breeds are especially prone to respiratory problems and they are usually the ones with short noses such as Pugs, Pekingese and Bulldogs for the obvious reason that a shorter nose has less of the body's defenses to deal with before getting to the lungs, these breeds tend to have problems of the upper respiratory tract. Other problem breeds for this system are Grey Hounds and Great Danes that are more predisposed to Pneumonia because of small or narrow thoracic space.

Rhinitis

The name means inflammation of the mucous membranes of the nose and usually appears as part of a disease or one of the symptoms of a disease. The inflammation process is usually started by some irritant factor and maybe opens the way for a secondary infection. The first sign that a dog has been infected with something is usually sneezing and a watery nose.

Signs and Symptoms

Usually a constant symptom that starts as a thin

discharge and gradually thickens and changes in quality. The discharge may be acrid in which case excoriation (burning) of the nostrils will soon be seen sometimes there may be blood in the discharge. When persistent mucopurulent discharges are present they may impede breathing by blocking the nostrils you can tell this by placing a finger in front of each nostril and feeling the breath.

Herbal Treatment

Always start treatment with Echinacea, Garlic and Vitamin C because we don't know what sort of problem may be developing and its best to always stop it at the start and if this is a worst case scenario then we have given it the best start. The main Action to look at here is those of the Anti-catarrhal Herbs with some good ones to consider being Elder and Eyebright especially when the eyes are watery. Consider also the Anti-inflammatory herbs and ones like Golden that do both.

Homoeopathic Treatment

Arsenic Album 30C- For the early stages when the discharge is thin and acrid, eyes my be watery and patient is thirsty for small quantities of water.

Allium Cepa 6C - Discharges are usually thin and watery accompanied by sneezing and watery eyes, useful in the first stages.

Kali Bich 6C - Yellow discharges which develop into small plugs which have a tough stringy appearance. Streaks of blood are often present.

Mercurius 6C - Greenish discharge, may contain

blood, nasal bones are frequently swollen.

Pulsatilla 30C- Mild tempered animals showing changeable moods, discharge thick and creamy, there may be ulceration with small streaks of blood.

Sinusitis

Inflammation of the sinus is usually the result of a infection. The pain is usually from the pressure the expanding mucous puts on the surrounding area. Infection usually spreads from other areas with a common cause being a infected tooth.

Signs and Symptoms

After a period of time the infection leads to a softening of the bone covering of the maxillary sinus and ulceration. Infection of a frontal sinus usually results in a purulent nasal discharge which becomes streaked with blood. There is usually accompanying conjunctivitis and pain over the sinus affected. The temperature may be raised. As for any health problem try to remove the cause, in this case it could be a infected tooth.

Herbal Treatment

With this condition we need to find the cause for treatment to be really effective. Some herbs to look at here are Ginger and Cayenne which are warm spicy circulatory stimulants which act by thinning the mucous and are called mucotropic. For this condition in its chronic state the herb to use is Fenugreek as this not only thins the mucous but it is also a lymphatic cleanser so it will start to slowly move all the rubbish out. The golden rule here is that for every year the condition has existed you will need at least one month of treatment. For the acute condition think of Garlic, Echinacea, Golden Rod and Eyebright if the eyes are affected. Actions to consider for this condition are Anti biotic, Anti catarrhal, Anti-inflammatory and if you believe that the mucus is burning or irritating the skin consider the Action of Demulcents and Emollients. I would also give a good dose of Vitamin C till the situation improves to help boost the immune system.

What usually happens in sinusitis is the trapped mucous increases leading to the bone aching pains of this condition which leads us to our next herb Wood Betony which is used for pains in the head and face.

Homoeopathic Treatment

Hepar Sulph 30C - Indicated where there is pain and sensitivity over the affected area. Low potencies will promote expulsion of any residual pus while high potencies will provide healing by granulation.

Silicea 30C - For long standing cases where symptoms are less sensitive. It will help the healing process by drying any discharge and removing scar tissue.

Tonsillitis

Inflammation can be acute or chronic and is fairly common. The affected tissue becomes swollen and reddened due to increased blood supply and may show small greyish spots of necrosis and frothy exudate. Appetite may be variable and there is discomfort on swallowing.

Signs and Symptoms

Reaching is a frequent accompaniment with vomiting of any excess mucous. A rise of temperature is usual in the early stages. There may be fever and there may also be enlarged lymph glands of the neck also look for difficulty in swallowing.

Herbal Treatment

Herbal Actions to think of here are those of the Anti-microbial Herbs such as Echinacea, Myrrh and Sage which is a specific for the throat area. Meaning as though the tonsils are part of the lymphatic system we should look at some herbs that have a affinity to this system especially in cleaning it with some good ones being Cleavers, Poke Root (use in very, very small doses) and think of Fenugreek for long term use upon recovery to clean out the system. Consider also the Anti-inflammatory to help with the pain along with the Demulcents to soothe or one that does both such as Licorice. Thyme is another good throat and mouth remedy.

Homoeopathic Treatment

Acute Form

Aconitum 6C - Give as early as possible where it can sometimes stop the problem from developing further.

Apis 6C - Excessive edema of tonsillar tissue, warm drinks aggravate.

Belladonna 30C - A useful remedy along with Aconitum in the early stages. The patient may show excitability with dilated pupils and a full throbbing pulse.

Merc Sol 6C - Lots of ropey saliva present together with ulceration of the gums and tonsil area.

Phytolacca 30C - Where the tonsils are enlarged and the throat has a dark red color. Membranous deposits may be present along with yellowish mucous.

Rhus Tox 6C - The throat shows large amounts of mucous and assumes a unnatural reddish color. Externally the throat may be swollen. There may be accompanying eye symptoms.

Chronic Form

This can be a sequel to some disease in the past that has not left the system yet, a good example could be distemper. The following remedies will be of help.

Baryta Carb - 6C - Both very young and old subjects will benefit from this remedy. There is a marked tendency to suppuration of the tonsillar tissue.

Hepar Sulph 30C - Tonsils which periodically show purulent infection may be helped by this remedy. The throat becomes extremely painful and sensitive to pressure during acute episodes.

Kali Bich 6C - Swollen tonsils becoming ulcerated and yielding a stringy yellow pus, the tissue assumes a reddish coppery tinge.

Silicea 30C - Promotes the absorption of any fibrous or scar tissue which may be present and will control and tendency to suppuration.

Streptococcus Nosode 30C - This nosode can be combined with the above remedies.

Laryngitis

Inflammation of the larynx may be acute or chronic. The acute form is usually associated with a primary infection or from another problem having spread. Some have attributed the condition to excessive or prolonged barking. The chronic form is characterized hypertrophy of laryngeal tissue often with a membranous deposit covering the larynx. It is associated with edema and swelling of the throat.

Signs and Symptoms

The quality of the bark becomes altered, a hoarse growl being emitted instead of the normal sound. Excessive mucous of a frothy nature is present. Pain could also be a factor along with swallowing. Check the neck glands for swelling.

Herbal Treatment

Treat this condition the same as tonsillitis and make good use of the main throat herbs Sage and Thyme.

Homoeopathic Treatment

Acute Form

Aconitum 6C - Give as early as possible where it can sometimes stop the problem from developing further.

Apis 30C - Much edema and throat swelling, aversion to warmth of any kind.

Belladonna 30C - Indicated for the animal which shows excitability, full bounding pulse and throbbing arteries, can be profitably combined with the above remedy.

Drosera 9C - Spasmodic cough associated with the

upper trachea and larynx, hoarseness is very pronounced, there is also tenacious mucous, the cough usually produces reaching and vomiting in the dog and greatly impedes breathing.

Spongia 6C - Indicated in laryngeal conditions attended by a hoarse croupous cough, there is a absence of mucous, there may be whistling with the respiration.

Chronic Form

Phytolacca 30C - Useful in those cases where a membranous deposit covers the affected area, marked redness of the larynx.

Silicea 30C - This remedy helps promote healing of fibrous tissue and will hasten absorption of scar tissue and guard against infection.

Cough

While coughing is frequently associated with various pulmonary infections it may arise as a seemingly independent syndrome and takes various forms. The main ones to consider besides the obvious are Distemper, Heart disease and Heart Worms, Lung worm, TB, Hepatitis and Round worms.

Various Types Of Cough

1/. Pleuritic cough - Short and dry and the animal shows pain while coughing.

2/. Bronchitic cough - Starts dry and frequent, becomes moist and soft.

3/. Simple catarrhal cough - Usually moist and infrequent.

4/. Pneumonic cough - Frequent, may contain rust colored fibrous deposits in the sputum.
5/. Stomach or intestinal cough - Various forms dependent on alimentary disorders.

Herbal Treatment

The herbal Actions to look at here are those of the Expectorants with licorice being one of the best, then look at the Anti-Catarrhal. If the cough is painful look at the Demulcents and Anti-Inflammatory. For a cough like Whooping cough which is spasmodic, painful and may sometimes stop the patient from getting a breath use Wild Cherry Bark as this suppresses the main respiratory nerve and should bring relief.

Kennel Cough - Tracheobronchitis

The term "Kennel Cough" is the common name used for Canine Infectious Tracheobronchitis also known as Bordetellosis, or Bordetella. This is a highly infectious airborne disease. The disease can last from 10-20 days. Kennel Cough is a upper respiratory disease caused by several different viruses and bacteria. In the majority of cases the disease is not serious in itself but it can lead to some dogs developing life threatening complications such as exudative pneumonia.

Signs and Symptoms

Coughing is a constant sign, the type of cough being described as hacking usually short in duration and dry in quality but occasionally a succession of short coughs develop which produce a paroxysmal effect. Light pressing on the trachea may induce the cough. The cough has been described as "as if something is caught in his throat" and also as Honking. Symptoms are confined to the upper respiratory area and systemic involvement is extremely uncommon. Other symptoms to look for are watery nose and or eyes discharge, fever, lethargy and wheezing.

Herbal Treatment

Start treatment with Echinacea, Garlic and Vitamin C. Because of the hoarseness of the cough use Expectorants that are Demulcent such as Licorice, Mullein and Plantain. If there is lots of mucous we need to use Astringents to slow the flow maybe Eye Bright (good for when the eyes are watering) and Elecampane (anti-bacterial to). If there is a fever consider the Diaphoretic herbs. Other actions to consider are Anti Inflammatory and Anti Catarrhal. Other herbs to look at are Coltsfoot, Golden Rod, Hyssop and Horehound with the last two being good for the cough. The herb Licorice covers actions needed for this condition. Rub some Eucalyptus oil into the throat.

Homoeopathic Treatment

Aconitum 6C - Should be given as early as possible in the infection where it will help allay development. It will also ease the condition by calming the animal and is especially useful in the evening for this purpose.

Bryonia 30C - The pleurae become involved when this remedy is indicated. Breathing becomes of the abdominal type because of the pain in the intercostal muscles. Pressure over or on the chest relieves the symptoms and the animal prefers rest.

Drosera 9C - Spasmodic cough associated with the upper trachea and larynx, hoarseness is very pronounced, there is also tenacious mucous, the cough usually produces reaching and vomiting in the dog and greatly impedes breathing.

Ipecacuanha 30C - Coughing produces reflex vomiting which can be frequent, cough is worse at night, cold atmosphere can excite cough, blood may show in the vomit and expectoration. Respiration has been described as sighing.

Phosphorus 30C - Indicated in dry cough with flecks of blood appearing in the nasal passages, the animal may show excitability, rapid breathing with threatened pneumonia may occur.

Rumex 6C - The cough is attended by much mucous and is relived in the evening or during the night, the character of the cough changes frequently

Spongia 6C - The cough is of the harsh dry variety, sometimes hoarse and a whistling sound may be present, can be associated with weak heart action.

Bronchiectasis

This is where the bronchial tree becomes abnormally dilated due to a loss of tone or elasticity in its fibres. This allows fluid to develop in pockets which eventually become pockets for purulent material along with airflow obstruction and impaired clearance of secretions. This condition is frequently a sequel to some other pulmonary disease but it can also arise as a result of a foreign body being breathed into the lung.

Signs and Symptoms

Continual coughing which is dry and unproductive in the early stages but soon becomes moist and the patient coughs up large quantities of mucopurulent material. Usually with this problem there are other things wrong or have been in the respiratory system, it would be a good idea to get a chest x-ray just to see exactly what's going on.

Herbal Treatment

Choose herb from the expectorants which you think best covers the symptoms. With this condition the long term use of Fenugreek is recommended for this will keep the mucous thin and non-sticky as well as being a tonic to the system. With this being a long term condition use Echinacea on a month on month off basis so as not to burn out the immune system. Calc Flour below is the most important remedy for this condition as even getting a little bit of elasticity back would improve the situation.

Homoeopathic Treatment

Antimonium Tart 30C - A useful remedy in the early stages when the cough is attended with frothy exudate.

Calc Flour 6X - This tissue salt helps put the elasticity back into muscles.

Hepar Sulph 30C - A good remedy in the early

purulent stages and will limit the risk of secondary bacterial involvement.

Kali Bich 30C - Indicated when the cough is accompanied by tough mucous of a yellow stringy nature.

Merc Sol 6C - This remedy could be indicated when any material coughed up is of a greenish rather than of a yellow color.

Chronic Bronchitis

This condition can be caused from a genetic weakness or as a result from acute conditions such as Kennel Cough leaving damage. The main causes are persistent low grade infections or irritations which slowly over time produce irreversible changes to the bronchi. In elderly dogs the condition may be from a weak heart.

Signs and Symptoms

In most cases the cough develops slowly and at first may only be present during exertion. Many cases will not develop further then this but a few do get worse and then it can turn into a very debilitating disease. There is a wet cough that can be excited by exercise and frequent movement. Rest seems to relieve the problem. There is usually a history of respiratory problems.

Herbal Treatment

The treatment is fairly much the same as Colds and Influenza but we concentrate on the Actions of the Expectorants, Anti Inflammatories and Demulcents especially when there are signs of pain with the cough. Here are a list of some other Herbs that are very good for the treatment of bronchitis - Coltsfoot, Elecampane, Horehound, Licorice, Mullein, Pleurisy Root and Horehound. If the cough is unproductive and causing pain think of Wild Cherry Bark which will act upon the nerve to stop the cough. Also consider boosting the immune system because raw and damaged mucous tracts are very prone to secondary infections. I would also give a large dose of Vitamin C every day.

Another thing we can do is to get a humidifier or something similar and put in one tablespoon of Eucalyptus oil and let it fill the room as Eucalyptus is a bronchodilator and this could give some relief. For the very chronic form of the disease especially in the old dog or where there might be heart problems think of giving the herb Astragalus on a regular basis, have a good look into this very important herb along with Hawthorn which can strengthen the heart beat thus reducing lung edema.

Homoeopathic Treatment

Antimonium Tart 30C - A useful remedy in the early stages when the cough is frequent and attended with frothy exudate.

Bryonia 30C - The pleurae become involved when this remedy is indicated. Breathing becomes of the abdominal type because of the pain in the intercostal muscles. Pressure over or on the chest relieves the symptoms and the animal prefers rest.

Dulcamara 6C - Condition has origins from damp surroundings and coughing worse after exertion.

Drosera 6C - Coughing becomes spasmodic in character, paroxysms follow one another rapidly.

Kali Bich 30C - Indicated when the cough is accompanied by tough mucous of a yellow stringy nature which the animal has a hard time bringing up.

Rumex 6C - The cough is attended by much mucous and is relived in the evening or during the night, the character of the cough changes frequently, this is also a good remedy for the heart.

Spongia 6C - The cough is of the harsh dry variety, sometimes hoarse and a whistling sound may be present, can be associated with weak heart action.

Diseases of the Lungs and Pleura

Pulmonary Edema

The abnormal accumulation of fluid in the lungs is usually a sequel to chronic heart disease, especially mitral valve insufficiency which causes weak circulation and allows fluid to gather in areas. Edema may also be a sequel to distemper.

Signs and Symptoms

There is great difficulty in breathing and a wet cough is fairly constant. Here you have to decide if this is a heart or respiratory problem. The age and case history should give you the clues needed.

Herbal Treatment

If this condition is caused by a failing heart the herbs to look at here are Hawthorn or Broom with

Hawthorn being the best but if it is from a infection treat as Pneumonia.

Homoeopathic Treatment

These are heart remedies look at Pneumonia for lung remedies.

Apis 30C - This remedy is always indicated when edema is present.

Adonis Vernalis 6C - This is also a good heart remedy which should have a beneficial effect in valvular disease.

Cactus Grandiflourus 6C - This is a good heart remedy which will stimulate the hearts action and thereby increase circulation.

Crataegus 6C - A heart remedy which exerts its action on the muscle thereby increasing the force of the beat and the flow of the circulation.

Carbo Veg 30C - Gives relief by helping the patient's oxygen supply and thereby aiding breathing in general.

Emphysema

When the alveoli of the lungs lose their elasticity becoming distended and unable to return to their normal size a state of emphysema is said to exist. In severe cases the alveolar wall may rupture permitting the escape of air into surrounding tissues. This condition is usually caused or is the end result of other diseases with a good example being pneumonia.

Signs and Symptoms

There is obvious difficulty in expelling air and respiration may be associated with forced movements of the abdominal muscles in order to assist the process. There is general difficulty in breathing. Tension in the pulmonary vessels arise as a result of increased pressure on the right ventricle of the heart.

Herbal Treatment

This is a long term chronic disease and treatment would be similar to what is mentioned in Bronchiectasis with the addition of Coltsfoot. With this condition the long term use of Fenugreek is recommended for this will keep the mucous thin and non-sticky as well as being a tonic to the system. Panax Ginseng Capsules could be useful by raising the life force and another one to look at is Astragalus, these to herbs are what is known as Adaptogens, they don't heal but they give energy and help the body to get the best out of what's left of it helping the patient to get the best out of their condition. In humans for this condition and for heart failure I have been using Co enzyme Q10 which is a new remedy which makes the body function better with low oxygen Try 50mg 3 times a day and see what happens..

Homoeopathic Treatment

These remedies will work at the onset of the condition but will not be much help in the chronic condition.

Acconitum 6C - Always indicated where there is tension in any part of the circulatory system and should give relief indirectly as a result.

Carbo Veg 30C - Will provide oxygen by its ability to help in cases of air hunger, will give relief particularly at night.

Lobellia 30C - Useful in the treatment of functional emphysema where the changes in the alveolar walls have not gone too far or become chronic.

Pneumonia

Inflammation of the lung tissue may appear as a result of exposure to cold and damp and also as a sequel to disease such as Bronchitis. Deficiencies of Calcium and Magnesium or these minerals out of balance can cause respiratory problems. Another cause can be by over rich unnatural diets which in turn clog the blood stream and cause excessive formations of mucous, the lungs having so much traffic with the blood stream they are made unhealthy. The Pus forming bacteria Pneumococci would not be present in large numbers unless there were sufficient mucous and toxic accumulations to nourish them that is why healthy animals don't usually get this problem. Pneumonia is basically inflammation of the air sacks of the lung with exudation and consolidation. X-ray usually confirms diagnosis.

Signs and Symptoms

There is an initial rise in temperature followed by a nasal discharge of muco-purulent material which may be streaked with blood. Respirations are increased and in severe cases painful breathing is evident.

Coughing is a fairly constant sign and if bacterial or viral invasion is thought to have taken place other systemic signs may appear such as vomiting or constipation. The animal becomes dehydrated and unkempt and water intake is decreased. A typical case may look like - breathing rapidly with mouth closed, eyes will be blood shot and there may be a high fever.

Herbal Treatment

Juliette de Bairacli would always start treatment for such a serious disease with a fast so as to rest the body and clean off the accumulated toxins. Next she uses the Antiseptic herbs such as Garlic and Eucalyptus. After this comes strengthening and soothing the body mainly with honey which could be rolled into balls on a board powdered with slippery elm and medicated with a few drops of Eucalyptus oil, add to this fresh air and Vitamin C. She would also let the fever run its course for this is nature's way of fighting the disease. Right lets stand back and see what she is doing. Fasting is always a good way of starting treatment as it takes the weight off the digestive system and gives the body time to cleanse, while all this is going on you get a chance to get a good look at all the symptoms and what's happening. Garlic is the most important herb in respiratory conditions as it is a Anti-Viral and Anti-Bacterial and always exits the body via the mucous membranes (hence Garlic Breath) and with the lungs being one of the biggest mucous membrane of the body we are putting our two actions just where we need them. Eucalyptus Oil could also be diluted with carrier oil and rubbed on tummy especially where it meets the chest as essential oils cross over to the blood stream where the Antiseptic action will be useful. Other herbs to think of are Echinacea as an immune booster, Elecampane for its Anti-Bacterial, Diaphoretic, Expectorant and soothing actions. If there seems to be pain add Mullein. The main actions to use here are Expectorants, Diaphoretics, Anti-Inflammatories and Anti-Catarrhals. Other herbs to look at are Golden Rod, Horehound, Coltsfoot, Hyssop, Plantain and Licorice.

Homoeopathic Treatment

The following remedies may help if the symptoms match.

Aconitum 6C - Give as early as possible where it can sometimes stop the problem from developing further.

Antimonium Tart 30C - Where there is a abundance of loose mucous and expectoration.

Bryonia 6C - When this remedy is indicated the animal resents movement, pressure over the affected area brings relief, the animal prefers to lie on the effected side.

Ferrum Phos 6C - The animal may show signs of pain and anxiety when breathing in. There is a abundance of loose mucous in the throat. Coughing may produce blood and is associated with blood.

Phosphorus 30C - Expectoration of rust colored sputum may accompany vomiting. Alternatively the cough may be dry and unproductive. A good remedy for nervous and sensitive animals.

Pleurisy

Inflammation of the pleural membranes can be either dry or accompanied by effusion into the pleural sack. The cause is usually from the spread of infection from another part of the respiratory system. Injuries to the chest may lead to pleurisy and it may also arise from exposure to cold and damp. This is a very painful condition.

Signs and Symptoms

The animal appears anxious and there are signs of abdominal breathing signifying pain on inspiration. If one side only is effected the animal seeks to lie on that side while if the animal assumes a sitting position it usually indicates both sides are effected. The temperature may rise to 105 F and accompanies early signs of pain.

Herbal Treatment

Pleurisy is a infection so we shall attack the infection directly with Echinacea and Garlic, fever can also be a large part of pleurisy so we will attack this symptom with the herbs that are called Diaphoretics which are herbs used for fevers, some of them are Yarrow, Peppermint and Elder. As there is a lot of pain with this condition we shall add some Demulcent (soothing Herbs) herbs which will hopefully sooth the effected membranes and reduce the pain, a good one here to use is Mullein and I would also be inclined to add Coltsfoot for its all-round effect. For the Anti-Inflammatory herbs it would be a tossup between Comfrey and Golden Rod as these are both good all round herbs and their actions cover most of the symptoms of this disease. Also have a good look at the herb called Pleurisy Root. So a possible good formula we could make would be Echinacea, Garlic, Mullein, Yarrow and Comfrey at about 20% each so it is easy to make up. Try to make your formulas no more than five herbs at a time and try to base them on the actions you need. Always consider the pain side of this condition as it can cause extreme pain.

Homoeopathic treatment

Acconitum 30C - Should always be given as early in the condition as possible, as it will quickly allay anxiety and helps to relieve pain.

Apis 30C - This remedy should help to reduce the fluid which is present in those cases showing effusion.

Belladonna 30C - A useful remedy if the animal feels unduly hot with dilated pupils and throbbing pulse.

Bryonia 6C or 30C - This is probably the best remedy to consider in most cases once the condition has established. A main guiding principle for its use is relief of pain on pressure seen by the animal lying on the effected side and disinclined to move.

Cantharis 200C - Pleural effusion, mucous expectorated with cough is usually blood stained, severe straining when trying to pass urine.

Kali Carb 200C - Symptoms of pain worse on right

side, cough worse in early morning and there is usually a dry throat. Dose 3 times daily for 3 days.

Sulphur 6C - Use in the convalescent stage of pleurisy. Dose once daily for 6 days.

Herbal Overview Of The Respiratory System

For most conditions of the respiratory system Echinacea and Garlic should be very seriously considered especially if the condition is a result of bacteria or viruses and even if it is not they should still be considered as a preventative for secondary infections. Doses of Vitamin C are also very important to consider. Licorice is another good herb for the respiratory system as some of its actions are expectorant and demulcent but the main reason I am mentioning it is that you usually add licorice to a herbal formula so as to help the body of the patient to absorb the formula. Try not to use more than five herbs in a formula and use the actions you require to select the herbs, you can do this easily by using my First Aid For Animals Booklet by accessing the Herbal and Actions section.

Below are the Actions to think of when dealing with the Respiratory System. As usual isolate the animal and observe. Consider also if the condition is effecting another system ?. Is there diarrhea, is there any unusual behavior, is there fever, what is the temperature, is the animal anxious etc. Some of the best herbs for this system are Angelica, Coltsfoot,

Comfrey, Elder, Elecampane, Eyebright, Fenugreek, Golden Rod, Hyssop, Horehound, Horse Radish, Licorice, Mullein, Myrrh, Plantain, Sage and Thyme.

Herbal Actions Of The Respiratory System

Anti-biotic - Echinacea, Elecampane, Garlic, Burdock, Myrrh.

Anti-catarrhal - Helps the body to remove excess catarrhal build ups.

Herbs - Cayenne, Coltsfoot, Cranesbill, Echinacea, Elder, Eyebright, Garlic, Golden Rod, Hyssop, Marshmallow, Mullein, Myrrh, Peppermint, Sage, Thyme, Yarrow.

Anti-inflammatory - Helps the body to combat inflammations. Herbs mentioned under demulcents will often act in this way especially when they coat sore throats and pipe lines.

Herbs - Comfrey, Cranesbill, Eyebright, Feverfew, Ginger, Golden Rod, Ladys Mantle, Licorice, Marshmallow.

Anti-microbial - Helps the body destroy or resist pathogenic micro-organisms.

Herbs - Aniseed, Echinacea, Garlic, Myrrh, Peppermint, Plantain, Rosemary, Sage, Thyme.

Antispasmodic - Prevents or eases spasms and cramps.

Herbs - Aniseed, Coltsfoot, Fennel, Horehound, Hyssop, Mullein, Rosemary, Sage, Skullcap, Thyme

Anti-viral - Astragalus, Echinacea, Elecampane, Garlic, Myrrh?, Shitake, St Johns Wort, Pau D'Arco.

Anthelmintic - Destroys or expels worms from the digestive system.

Herbs - Garlic, Tansy, Wormwood, Thyme, Rue.

Astringent - Contracts tissue which in turn reduces discharges, these herbs contain tannins.

Herbs - Agrimony, Comfrey, Elecampane, Eyebright, Golden Rod, Marshmallow, Mullein, Myrrh, Plantain, Sage, Rosemary, Shepherds Purse, Thyme.

Demulcent - Soothes and protects irritated or inflamed internal tissues.

Herbs - Coltsfoot, Comfrey, Fenugreek, Licorice, Marshmallow, Mullein, Oats, Plantain.

Diaphoretic - Aids the skin in the elimination of toxins and produces sweat thus reducing the temperature of fevers.

Herbs - Cayenne, Elder, Elecampane, Fennel, Garlic, Ginger, Golden Rod, Hyssop, Peppermint, Thyme, Yarrow.

Expectorant - Supports the body in the removal of excess mucous from the respiratory system and helps in the control of coughs.

Herbs - Aniseed, Coltsfoot, Comfrey, Elder, Elecampane, Fennel, Fenugreek, Garlic, Hyssop, Horehound, Licorice, Marshmallow, Mullein, Myrrh, Plantain, Sweet Violets, Thyme.

Febrifuge - Helps the body to bring down fevers.

Herbs - Cayenne, Elder Flowers, Hyssop, Marigold, Penny Royal, Peppermint, Plantain, Raspberry, Sage, Thyme, Vervain.

Immune Booster - Astragalus, Echinacea, Reshi, Shitake.

Pectoral - Has a general strengthening and healing effect on the respiratory system.

Herbs - Aniseed, Coltsfoot, Comfrey, Elder, Garlic, Hyssop, Licorice, Mullein, Horehound.

Notes

The Digestive System

Diarrhea and Constipation

Character of the Stools

Stools may be watery, mucous or dysenteric with varying degrees of color and consistency. Large evacuations indicate that the source of the trouble is in the small intestines while small stools frequently evacuated may indicate colitis as does the presence of a large amount of mucous. Frothy stools which may contain fat globules frequently indicate pancreatitis or diabetes. Black stools indicate bleeding somewhere in the intestinal tract. Clay colored stools are associated with liver and bile dysfunction while the presence of orange pigment usually means that a leptospiral infection is present.

Herbal Treatment

Diarrhea

This is a method the body uses to get rid of toxins that are aggravating it so it is best to let it run its course and be on the watch for dehydration and take steps to prevent this from happening. Some people give laxatives with this condition so as to try to clear the toxins out fast. Always try to find the cause of the problem, is it diet, stress, allergies etc. Gastritis is a common cause for diarrhea followed by worm infestations or it could be part of a symptom picture of a infectious disease. The dog should be fasted till the condition improves or for 24 hours at least. Diarrhea is usually treated with Astringents usually the milder ones as the very strong ones may upset a sensitive tummy. Some examples are Agrimony, Meadowsweet and Slippery Elm which is the best for recovery as it is Demulcent and Nutritive. If a infectious type of disease is suspected add Garlic and Echinacea. Usually with the more serious diseases there is a rise in the temperature.

Constipation

Can be mild or severe and has its origin in reduced fluid intake, poor diet, the consumption of large amounts of bones, anal sack problems or sometimes just old age. The first place to start is to look at the diet.

Laxative herbs are Burdock, Dandelion, Licorice, Fumitory and Horseradish. Stronger ones are Cascara and Senna Pods.

Homoeopathic Treatment

Diarrhoea - Use the remedies listed in Enteritis and Colitis in the Homoeopathic Section.

Constipation

Can be mild or severe and has its origin in reduced fluid intake, the consumption of large amounts of bones or sometimes just age.

Nux Vom 1M - There is frequent straining with passage of small amounts at a time. The origin of the trouble is usually dietary upset and may be associated with vomiting. This is a good digestive remedy and will help regulate proper bowel movements.

Sulphur 6C - Usually pronounced redness around the anus accompanied by much scratching in general, body odor may be musty, acts well with Nux Vom.

Bryonia 6C - Stools are large and dark colored and passed more frequently in the morning, the animal is generally uneasy and is disinclined to move. Tenderness over the abdomen is very pronounced although pressure is not resented.

Lycopodium 1M - Usually a history of liver problems or accompanying hepatitis. Stools are small and the appetite is capricious, very little satisfying. Lean or undernourished looking animals may respond well to this remedy with other symptoms agreeing.

Gastritis (Acute)

Inflammation of the stomach is common and is usually due to irritants of one form or another. Gastritis can also be a sequel or accompaniment to acute infectious diseases such as Hepatitis and Leptospirosis. Dogs eating grass is an instinctive process and can be a sign of stomach problems. Grass eating can be just a simple habit or possibly the sign of a stomach irritation such as Gastritis. Eating grass can stimulate or induce vomiting. Grass can in fact help to prevent damage to the bowel as grass is effective in wrapping around any foreign bodies in the stomach thus limiting the risk of damage to the stomach form any sharp or jagged edges.

Signs and Symptoms

There is usually constant thirst and vomiting with a temperature rise if the condition is associated with a infectious disease. Pain on palpation of the stomach area is usually present. Signs of dehydration quickly set in especially if vomiting is severe or prolonged and is worse in puppies and young animals. A short fast for 24 hours would allow the situation to settle and give you time to see if the condition is getting better or worse. Always try to find the cause, what's the dog been eating? is the temperature rising if so it may be an infectious disease.

Herbal Treatment

The main herbal Actions we need to look at for this condition are the Anti-Inflammatorys and the Demulcents. Marshmallow, Slippery Elm and Comfrey are soothing Demulcent herbs which should line and sooth the raw areas while Meadowsweet will deal with the inflammation and pain etc. Other herbs to look at are Peppermint, Fennel and Licorice.

Homoeopathic Treatment

Phosphorus 30C - Pronounced thirst but vomiting takes place as soon as the contents of the stomach become warm after drinking, gums may be ulcerated with slight bleeding, stools may be clay colored.

Ipecacuanha 30C - Retching and vomiting may lead to collapse. The vomit is slimy and may be continuous. Slimy diarrhea possibly blood stained may be present also. There may also be reflex respiratory symptoms such as coughing and difficulty in breathing.

Antimonium Tart 30C - The tongue is coated with red edges, swallowing is difficult and is accompanied by retching and vomiting, rumbling of intestines may be heard preceding stool which is accompanied by straining, the stools themselves being watery with shreds of mucous.

Arsen Alb 30C - Mouth is ulcerated and dry, thirst is prominent but there is a desire for small quantities only. Blood may be in the vomit, the animal is usually restless changing position frequently and all symptoms become worse toward and after midnight. The coat is dry and harsh.

Iodum 30C - This remedy may be suitable for the lean animal showing cadaverous hunger with diarrhea of a pale frothy character, mouth and tongue may show ulcers, liver complications are a common feature with signs of jaundice.

Iris Vers 30C - Vomiting of biliary material accompanies colic and diarrhea with tenderness over the liver region, signs of jaundice may appear, useful remedy if gastritis and vomiting are thought to occur from liver or pancreatic dysfunction.

Petroleum 6C - Vomit is sour smelling, water accumulates readily in the mouth, passage of stool is followed by hunger which relieves temporarily. Diarrhea is watery and confined to daylight hours.

Nux Vom 6C - Stools are generally hard when this remedy is needed, gastritis is usually due to overeating especially of rich and unsuitable food.

Enteritis and Colitis

Enteritis and Colitis are inflammatory conditions of the intestines that usually result in diarrhea and or dysentery with the character of the stool varying considerably. Acute episodes may arise as a result of bacterial attack or may be from specific diseases such as Distemper, Leptospirosis etc., another cause could be through faulty feeding, indigestion and decomposing food. Always withhold food for 24 hours and see what happens, most of the time the problem sorts itself out.

Signs and Symptoms

Vomiting may be seen initially but the main symptom is diarrhea which at times may have blood in it. Temperature may arise if the attack is due to bacterial invasion but if poisoning is suspected the temperature will be normal. Pain is evident on abdominal palpation and rumbling of gut may be heard in the large bowel. Signs of dehydration appear if the diarrhea is prolonged.

Herbal Treatment

The main Herbal Actions to look at here are Anti-Inflammatorys, Demulcents and Astringents for the relief of diarrhea. Slippery Elm should be thought of here not just for its soothing Demulcent properties but because it is also astringent so it will help with diarrhea, Comfrey has similar actions, Marshmallow is another good Demulcent. Other herbs to look at are Agrimony, Cranesbill (astringent), Fennel, Chamomile, Meadowsweet, Licorice and Wild Yam for the inflammation and especially if there is abdominal any pain. Think of Echinacea and Garlic if you think the cause is from a infection. For Puppies try to use mainly Agrimony and Chamomile, with a bit of Meadowsweet. Slippery elm is the main herb for the young for the reasons mentioned above and also because it is a nutritive herb and if mixed with a bit of raw honey you would increase the nutrition and supply a Antibiotic Action.

Homoeopathic Treatment

Arsen Alb 6 of 30C - This remedy is associated with watery stools of a cadaverous odor frequently worse in the evenings and towards midnight. Thirst for small amounts of water, the coat is harsh and dry and the patient is restless changing position from time to time, a good remedy when there are signs of dehydration.

Ipecac 30C - Indicated when severe vomiting precedes a attack, frequent mucous like stools which are greenish in color and may also be tinged with blood.

Podophyllum 30C - Remedy for conditions affecting both small and large intestines resulting in a gushing type of watery stool that may contain mucous. It is suitable for long standing diarrhea and may be accompanied by a degree of rectal prolapse.

Veratrum Alb 30C - Prostration accompanies the diarrhea and there is a general picture of collapse, signs of colic precede the onset of diarrhea which is profuse and watery. General signs include a dry mouth and cyanosis of visible mucous membranes.

Cuprum Met 30C - Muscular cramping may be seen accompanying diarrhea of a greenish blood stained character. Nervous symptoms are often present e.g twitching.

Carbo Veg 200C - A most useful remedy for the dead looking animal and will frequently give dramatic results in apparently hopeless cases which have suffered severe fluid loss. The stools have a cadaverous odour and are attended with considerable wind.

China 6C - This remedy should always be given as a accompaniment to others as it will help restore health after loss of body fluid, by itself it may control the diarrhea.

Aconitum 6C - Although not generally used as a remedy for diarrhea as such, this remedy should be given as soon as symptoms of illness arise, especially in the case of a specific disease.

Chronic Enteritis and Colitis

The main symptom is a chronic diarrhea which may be caused by the presence of foreign bodies or worms. The effects of tumor formation and pancreatic or liver disease may also contribute to it. Other causes include kidney diseases and nervous upsets.

Signs and Symptoms

Stools become mucoid with blood in them from time to time, there is a progressive loss of condition accompanying dehydration.

Herbal Treatment

Here we have to try and find the cause, use mainly the remedies in the acute condition section. If the cause is from worms look at Garlic, Tansy and Worm Wood though be careful of using strong herbs on a sensitive poorly system. If the problem is from tumors think of Burdock. If the problem is from the liver think of Milk Thistle. Consider a long fast at the beginning of the treatment so as to clean and give the system a break and latter start with lots of Slippery Elm and gentle herbs like Agrimony and Chamomile.

Homoeopathic Treatment

The remedies used in the acute condition can also be used in the chronic condition.

Ulcerative Colitis

This particular form of colitis is usually confined to young animals, especially those up to two years old. The Boxer breed is particularly susceptible. Mild cases can respond to dietary treatment alone.

Signs and Symptoms

The general condition of the animal remains good and the only important sign is the passage of soft stools containing a lot of mucous and showing streaks of blood. The character of the stool varies and is passed frequently, the color being a light brown. Sometimes the symptoms can go loose bowel then solid and keep going in that order especially if the dog has a nervous disposition.

Herbal Treatment

Many of the herbs under Enteritis and Colitis can be used especially the Anti-inflammatorys. Use lots of Demulcents like Slippery Elm and Marshmallow to sooth the irritated lining and if the cause is from a nervous origin, stress or even if it's just a nervy type of dog add some Nervines especially the ones that have actions on the nerves and digestive system such as Chamomile, Peppermint and another one to think of is Vervain. In this condition it is wise to use some Echinacea and Garlic because the ulceration will allow bowel bacteria to escape via the blood stream into other areas of the body and these herbs could help prevent complications. Remember to use Echinacea on a month on month off basis.

Homoeopathic Treatment

Many of the remedies under Enteritis and Colitis can be used if the diarrhea matches in addition to the remedies below.

Nitricum Acid 200C - This remedy is particularly suitable when ulceration of mucous membranes occurs near the outlet of natural orifices, and will therefore be indicated for those cases which develop lesions in the rectum as a extension from the colon.

Kali Bich 200C - A remedy for when the stools become jelly like and are passed more frequently in the mornings. Severe straining may accompany the passage of the stool and dysentery is often present.

Iodum 6C - When stools become frothy and yellow and are accompanied by voracious appetite and loss of condition, the skin has a dehydrated look.

Chamomilla 6C - Useful remedy for controlling diarrhea associated with upsets in the young animal, stools are hot and slimy and excoriate the skin around the anus.

Pancreatitis

This disease can start off acute and can then change into a chronic condition so great care must be taken to resolve this condition in its acute form. The causes are not really known but the diet should be checked for anything obvious. Some known causes are trauma and drugs. The pancreas is important for two of its main functions with the first being the control of carbohydrate metabolism through the use of insulin and the second being the production of enzymes which help to digest protein and fat. In a worst case the pancreas is basically being digested in its own enzymes.

Signs and Symptoms

Pancreatitis is inflammation of the pancreas which can be acute or chronic. The acute form is often seen in the over fat dog which has been fed a unbalanced diet of low protein and high fat though lean animals can be affected to. Arching of the back is a common sign and the abdominal muscles become hard. Attacks may come on suddenly and give rise to a state of shock. Temperature is at first raised but in severe cases tends to fall producing coldness of the body surface. Vomiting is usually severe and if not checked leads to dehydration. Pressure on the abdomen elicits pain. Stools are frothy and may contain fat globules. Increased thirst is evident. In others there can be anorexia, vomiting, weakness, abdominal pain, dehydration and diarrhea. In severe cases there will be shock.

Herbal Treatment

This is a hard one to treat and would be best to start with a fast for at least 3 to 4 days and see what happens from there. Some of the main herbs for this condition are Fringe Tree Bark and Fennel. Select herbs for the digestive system from the Anti-Inflammatories so as to help with the inflammation, consider also that this condition causes a lot of pain so think of herbs like Wild Yam and Demulcents like Licorice which may be of some use in soothing the irritated areas but is also good for inflammation and colic like pain. Consider also the liver as blocked bile duct can upset the pancreas next door so look at the Chologogues. Look at the diet to try and find the cause. If this is a chronic condition you may have to give digestive enzymes to help with the digestion. Try to look at the condition holistically and make a herbal formula that covers this.

Homoeopathic Treatment

Aconitum 12X - Suitable for the attack that comes on suddenly and will be indicated in the early high temperature stage.

Apocynum Cann 30C - Dropiscal conditions especially ascites (edema of the abdomen). Marked thirst and there may be excessive vomiting.

Apis 30C - Think of this remedy for edema and pain.

Colocynthis 30C - The back is arched from the pain, severe abdominal pain.

Iris Vers 30C - This is one of the most important remedies, vomiting may contain bile and stools become watery and greenish, abdominal pain is severe.

Iodium 6C - Stools are consistently frothy and fatty when this remedy is indicated. Suitable for the lean animal which shows a voracious appetite and dry coat, jaundice may be present.

Pancreas 30C - This is the pancreas nosode and it can be used along with the other remedies.

The Liver
Diseases of the Liver

Conditions affecting the functions of the liver may be caused from bacterial or viral infection or sometimes by a metabolic upset from faulty nutrition leading to as a example gallstones.

Signs and Symptoms

Palpation over the right abdominal area may reveal an enlarged liver which is not always associated with pain. Vomiting and lack of appetite are usually present with liver problems.

The color of the stool is a good guide to liver problems as the faeces can be orange or clay colored. Jaundice is a sign that the liver is not functioning as it should and can usually be seen as a yellowish color in the mucous membranes or the white parts of the eyes, with this sign there can also be bile in the urine giving it a yellowish greenish color. In chronic disease and those associated with tumor formation abdominal dropsy is usually present.

Herbal Treatment

With liver problems the best way to start would be a long fast so as to rest the liver and give it a chance to sort itself out. Finding the cause is most important as if it is infection you will need to give Echinacea and Garlic to start on the battle with the causative agents. Dandelion and Milk Thistle are the two main herbs to look at for serious liver problems other herbs to look at are listed under Hepatics - Gentian, Wormwood and Cholagogues - Agrimony, Fumitory.

Homoeopathic Treatment

This will depend on the overall symptom picture but there are certain remedies that have a action on the liver and they include the following

Chelidonium 6C - Yellowish tongue and discoloration of visible mucous membranes, vomiting is usually present and signs of stiffness or pain may be evident over the right shoulder region , stools are clay colored.

Phosphorus 200C - Vomiting is noticed shortly after animal takes food or water eg when it becomes warm in the stomach, small hemorrhages may be seen on the gums. With hepatitis the stools become pale and hard, the region over the liver becomes extremely tender on palpation.

Aesculus 30C - Jaundice, the portal circulation becomes congested leading to signs of abdominal discomfort soon after eating, tenderness over the liver, stools are large and hard and the urine becomes discolored, there may be accompanying respiratory symptoms such as coughing up mucous.

Lycopodium 1M- A prominent liver remedy, inability to eat much at any one time, very little food appears to satisfy, all symptoms aggravated in the late afternoon and early evening, a good remedy for the old and for lean animals, premature graying of the coat could be another sign for this remedy, stools are generally hard.

Nux Vom 1M - If liver dysfunction is secondary to overeating or partaking of unsuitable food this remedy will be indicated stools are hard and the animal's temperament becomes uncertain.

Sulphur 200C - For liver disturbances in dogs which show a dirty skin with redness of the skin around the anus and have a generally musty odor.

Infectious Canine Hepatitis

This is a worldwide viral infection spread by ingestion and is highly contagious, it may run a mild course which is hardly noticeable or be a severe infection with about 10% mortality. This infection can survive outside the host for months but can be killed by scrubbing suspected areas with household bleach. Animals that recover from this condition keep on passing the virus on through their urine for many months. This disease is also seen in foxes, wolves, coyotes and bears. Ingestion of urine, feces, or saliva of infected dogs is the main route of infection. Recovered dogs shed virus in their urine for more than 6 months.

Signs and Symptoms

The virus can affect all ages and has a incubation period of 10 days after which a rise in temperature occurs which subsides after one or two days and then rises again over a period of 5 to 6 days. Mild cases may show no other symptoms. If the disease progresses loss of appetite occurs along with increased thirst. Visible oral mucous membranes become congested having a reddish pink or red brick colored look. Small hemorrhages may appear on these membranes. Sometimes the throat becomes tender and swollen due to tonsillitis. The eyes are frequently affected with conditions ranging from lachrymation to conjunctivitis accompanying serous discharges. Edema of parts may be present, liver involvement is common giving rise to pain on palpation. Small hemorrhages of the skin occur in some cases mainly on the abdomen, if the dog injuries themselves while they are ill you will notice they bleed profusely and it is difficult to stop (Calendula Tincture externally on wound). Clotting time is directly correlated with the severity of illness.

Convalescent animals show weight loss which tends to persist even after the appetite returns to normal. On recovery, dogs eat well but regain weight slowly.

Herbal Treatment

With infectious diseases as fast acting and as serious as this use high doses of Vitamin C immediately, if you have it in liquid form such as Troys a 8cc dose intramuscularly should be given for the average size dog if not you can give it in Sodium Ascorbate Powder form at about 10 grams a day for the medium sized dog, you can mix the powder with water and gently syringe the liquid into the dogs mouth 3 times a day. It would be best to fast the dog especially at the beginning stages and it is not wise to give a dog food while they have a fever so try to wait till the fever breaks, meanwhile you could give the dog honey and water so they remain hydrated and have some nutrition. Use the immune boosting herbs Echinacea, Garlic and Myrrh constantly throughout the illness and add to them other herbs as the symptoms change. Try to match herbs to the symptoms being displayed like for the throat you could use Sage and Thyme (which can also be used for liver inflammation) for the liver problems we could use Dandelion, Fringe Tree Bark though Milk Thistle would be probably be better. Look to the Astringents for help for the bleeding with a good one internally being Shepherds Purse while Eye Bright could be used if the eyes were affected. Choose herbs from the Hepatics and Cholagogues but try to use ones that cover lots of actions you need.

Homoeopathic Treatment

Aconitum 30C - Should be given as soon as possible, one dose every hour for four doses, use this remedy for the sudden onset of any acute disease.

Crotalus Horr 30C - Probably the best remedy to give where stimulation of liver function is needed and bleedings show little signs of clotting.

Lachesis 30C - There is a strong tendency to hemorrhage and sepsis with profound prostration, it is particularly valuable if the throat develops inflammation causing left sided swelling that may involve a parotoid gland, where hemorrhage takes place the blood is dark and does not clot readily while the skin surrounding any lesion assumes a purplish appearance.

Phytolacca 30C - Throat symptoms should be relieved by this remedy especially cases showing enlargement of surrounding lymph glands.

Phoshorus 30C - The remedy of choice to control petechial and ecchymotic hemorrhages on the skin, it may also have a beneficial effect on the liver.

Rhus Tox 6X - A very useful remedy for the stage of mucous membrane involvement showing reddish discoloration, the eyes will also benefit from this remedy.

Hepatitis Nosode 30C - This can be given in conjunction with the other mentioned remedies and speed up the healing and gaining of weight.

Herbal Overview Of The Digestive System

Unfortunately one of the main ways of diagnosing what sort of disease a animal has is to do a autopsy straight after it has died, this has to be done especially in fast acting diseases that kill fast. Always isolate the animal from the others and clean and disinfect where the animal has been so as to minimize the spread of infection. In dealing with problems of the digestive system its always best to start with a purge so as to clean the system and bowels out. This is very important especially when you do not know what you are dealing with because you are purging out hopefully most of the toxins that are causing the condition. After the purge isolate and fast the animal for 24 hours and see what happens. Always start on the Garlic and Echinacea straight away as the Echinacea is also used to treat septicemia and to attack blood borne toxins and with Garlic being antiviral and antibacterial we have together a good strong initial attack . If you look at the herbal treatment sections above you will see they cover most of the conditions of the digestive system and should give you helpful information.

Below are a list of Herbal Actions that are used for the digestive system read through them and become familiar with them for in Herbal Medicine you always think in actions needed not the Herb needed this way the mind stays on the big picture.

Herbal Actions For The Digestive System

Anti-biotic - Always start with Garlic as this is both anti-bacterial and anti-viral as well as being used for killing parasites and worms, your initial attack begins here.

Herbs - Echinacea, Garlic, Myrrh, Pau D' Arco, Reshi.

Anti-emetic - Can reduce a feeling of nausea and can help to relieve or prevent vomiting.

Herbs - Cayenne, Fennel, Meadowsweet, Peppermint.

Anti-inflammatory - Helps the body to combat inflammations, there will always be pain, heat and maybe fever when these are called for. Herbs mentioned under demulcents will often act in this way especially when they are applied to coat for example a inflamed intestine or any other inflamed organ.(Slippery Elm).

Herbs - Cranesbill, Chamomile, Eyebright, Fennel, Feverfew, Ginger, Golden Rod, Ladys Mantle, Licorice, Marshmallow, Meadowsweet, Marigold, Pau D' Arco, Witch Hazel, Wormwood.

Anti-microbial - Helps the body destroy or resist pathogenic micro-organisms.

Herbs - Aniseed, Cayenne, Echinacea, Garlic, Gentian, Marigold, Myrrh, Peppermint, Rosemary, Rue, Sage, Thyme, Wormwood.

Antispasmodic - Prevents or eases spasms and cramps especially of the intestines.

Herbs - Aniseed, Angelica, Chamomile, Fennel, Rosemary, Rue, Sage, Skullcap, St Johns Wort, Thyme, Valerian, Vervain.

Anti-viral - Astragalus, Cats claw, Echinacea, Garlic, Myrrh?, Shitake, St Johns Wort, Pau D'Arco.

Anthelmintic - Destroys or expels worms from the digestive system.

Herbs - Garlic, Tansy, Wormwood, Thyme, Rue.

Aperient - Mild laxative.

Herbs - Burdock, Dandelion.

Astringent - Contracts tissue which in turn reduces discharges, these herbs contain tannins. In the digestive system they can be used to stop diarrhea and in the treatment of ulcers. Most astringents also have a anti-bacterial action.

Herbs - Agrimony, Bear Berry, Cranesbill, Comfrey, Eyebright, Golden Rod, Hops, Ladys Mantle, Marigold, Marshmallow, Meadowsweet, Nettles, Raspberry, Sage, Rosemary, Slippery Elm, Shepherds Purse, St Johns Wort, Slippery Elm, Thyme, Witch Hazel, Yarrow.

Bitters - Herbs that taste bitter act as stimulating tonics for the digestive system.

Herbs -Burdock, Feverfew, Gentian, Hops, Horehound, Rue, Tansy, Wormwood.

Carminative - Stimulates peristalsis of the digestive system and relaxes the stomach and helps remove gas and wind from the system. These herbs are usually rich in volatile oils.

Herbs - Aniseed, Angelica, Cayenne, Chamomile, Fennel, Garlic, Ginger, Golden Rod, Hyssop, Horseradish, Juniper, Parsley, Peppermint, Penny Royal, Sage, Rosemary, Tansy, Thyme, Valerian, Wormwood.

Cholagogue - Stimulates the release of bile from the gallbladder which can relieve gallbladder problems, bile is also the body's natural laxative so cholagogues have a laxative effect as well.

Herbs - Agrimony, Blue Flag, Dandelion, Fumitory, Gentian, Marigold, Milk Thistle, Yellow Dock.

Demulcent - Soothes and protects irritated or inflamed internal tissues.

Herbs - Bear Berry, Corn Silk, Coltsfoot, Comfrey, Fenugreek, Licorice, Marshmallow, Milk Thistle, Mullein, Oats, Plantain, Slippery Elm.

Diaphoretic - Aids the skin in the elimination of toxins and produces sweat thus reducing the temperature of fevers.

Herbs - Angelica, Black Cohosh, Cayenne, Chamomile, Elder, Elecampane, Fennel, Garlic, Ginger, Golden Rod, Guaiacum, Hyssop, Lime Blossom, Peppermint, Sarsaparilla, Thyme, Vervain, Yarrow.

Hepatic - Tones and strengthens the liver, may increase the flow of bile.

Herbs - Agrimony, Blue Flag, Dandelion, Fennel, Fumitory, Gentian, Horseradish, Hyssop, Motherwort, Milk Thistle, Vervain, Wormwood, Yarrow.

Laxative - Promotes the evacuation of the bowels.

Herbs - Burdock, Dandelion., Fumitory, Horseradish, Licorice.

Parasiticide - Kills parasites and insects.

Herbs - Aniseed, Rosemary.

Sialagogue - Stimulates the secretion of saliva.

Herbs - Blue flag, Cayenne, Gentian, Ginger.

Notes

The Nervous System

Epilepsy

This has no known cause but does occur more often in certain breeds such as the German shepherd and the Golden Retriever so the condition is probably hereditary. The first fit usually occurs when the dog is one or two years old and then tend to increase in frequency. Diagnosis is based on the breed, age and eliminating any other causes.

Signs and Symptoms

These may start off as minor convulsions which last sometimes less than a minute and usually do not have a loss of consciousness with them. These attacks tend to become more serious but less frequent as the animal gets older. Seizures are usually described in two forms the first being Petit Mal which is the milder version where the dog may simply develop a blank stare, or shake one leg or simply cry out as if in pain. The seizure is usually less than one minute. Grand Mal is the most common and the symptoms are falling to one side, they may urinate or defecate uncontrollably, paddle the feet as in swimming, froth at the mouth and they may also cry out. The patient may be unaware of their surroundings. With both kinds attacks can come on suddenly without any symptoms or there may be symptoms of restlessness or uneasiness prior to the seizure, afterwards the animal may be lethargic and sleepy looking.

Herbal Treatment

You need to try to prescribe on the whole picture of the dog and it may be worthwhile adding oats to the diet as this is a good nerve food or as it is properly called a Nervine Restorative. Herbs that have been used for epilepsy are Skullcap which is pretty much the specific, others to consider are Mistletoe, Gotu Kola, Hyssop, Vervain and Passion Flower. To build up the nervous system and strengthen it think of Oats, Chamomile and Valerian. The herbal actions we are mainly looking at are those of the Sedatives. If the dog is old and the condition is getting worse think of Ginkgo Biloba which will increase the blood supply to the head and maybe add to this Bacopa. Another herb I use as a last resort for this which is also used for dizzy spells and tinnitus is Black Cohosh, not because of its female actions as it is commonly used for but because it is a blood cleanser focused on the nervous system, I use this for 3 months as this is the blood cycle in the hope of cleaning out all the rubbish.

Homoeopathic Treatment

Belladonna 30C - This is one of the most frequently indicated remedies, for attacks associated with dilated pupils and throbbing pulse, the animal will usually feel abnormally hot.

Cocculus 6C - The main use for this remedy lies more in the preventative sphere and is useful to ward off subsequent attacks. It should be given at regular intervals over a period of a few months.

Cuprum Met 30C - A useful remedy when

convulsions are associated more with meningitis then with encephalitis. The head usually assumes a lowered posture and there may be attempts to press it against any suitable object.

Ignatia 6C - Consciousness is usually lost when this remedy is indicated. The head may be shaken to and fro and this precedes hysterical turns.

Hyoscyamus 30C - Indicated when attacks are preceded by shaking of the head and a unsteadiness of gait indicating vertigo, there may be spasmodic closing of the eyelid and the mouth is flecked with foam.

Stramonium 30C - This remedy is somewhat similar to the last one but there are usually signs before the fit such as staggering with a tendency to fall toward the left side, eyes are again dilated and staring.

Encephalitis

Encephalitis means infection of the brain. The main causes are viruses and bacteria of different kinds and some strains of Streptococci. Bacterial spreading from neighboring infected areas such as sinuses and eyes and ears can also lead to encephalitis. Some diseases that spread along the nervous system and may reach the brain are Rabies, Distemper, Parvovirus and Rocky Mountain Spotted Fever.

Signs and Symptoms

Symptoms can vary greatly depending on the cause but there may be varying degrees of nervous excitement seen in mild cases leading in more severe cases to convulsions. The eyes are usually staring and have a anxious or wild expression. The conjunctivae are red, facial twitching and head shaking may be present, the animal may cry out in pain, there is a staggering gait with stumbling and a tendency to fall forwards or backwards. There may be fever, confusion, vomiting, blindness and sometimes convulsions.

Herbal Treatment

Herbal treatment could be too slow for a fast acting disease as this but consider Garlic ,Echinacea and Myrrh for bacterial and viral infections. Essential oils can cross the blood brain barrier and could be a fast way of getting into the area so try maybe Garlic oil ,Lavender oil, Myrrh, Thyme or Eucalyptus diluted and rubbed in the area as these are all anti microbials. I have not heard of essential oils being used for this condition but as a last desperate resort I would try it. Homoeopathy is the better action to take as it is faster acting then herbal medicine.

Homoeopathic Treatment

Belladonna 30C - This is one of the chief remedies for relieving convulsions in the acute stage. Indications for its use are dilated pupils, throbbing pulse and redness of eyes.

Aconitum 30C - If attacks come on suddenly this remedy will help allay shock and limit the scope of the attack; it should be alternated every half hour with the previous remedy for a total of four doses each.

Stramonium 30C - This remedy may be useful for the less acute case which shows a staggering gait with a tendency to fall towards the left side or even backwards. Abdominal symptoms such as colic and diarrhea may accompany these attacks. Convulsive movements of the head are present and sight is usually lost.

Conium Mac 30C - Useful in the older animal, weakness of different kinds in the hind legs ranging from unsteady gait to a inability to rise with a progressive upwards paralysis.

Meningitis

This condition may be associated with encephalitis or arises independently and is usually associated with bacteria or viruses. This can be a very fast acting disease and is very similar to encephalitis.

Signs and Symptoms

The dog is usually more aware of its surroundings and reacts to external stimuli more noticeably then in a normal animal. The temperature is raised and the neck muscles become rigid causing the patient to keep the head in a fixed position rather than lower or raise it which appears to cause aggravation. This symptom is the main one pointing to meningitis.

Herbal Treatment

See herbal treatment in encephalitis, fast acting diseases like this may need fast acting drugs to bring the dog back from the brink.

Homoeopathic Treatment

Aconitum 6C - This remedy should be given as soon as the condition is noticed as it may stop or lessen further progress.

Stramonium 30C - Where there is a tendency to fall to one side mainly the left, abdominal symptoms such as colic and diarrhea may accompany these attacks and sight is usually diminished.

Belladonna 30C - Convulsive fits accompanied by foaming at the mouth, throbbing pulses and redness of the eyes, pupils are dilated and the animal feels hot all over.

Myelitis

This term means inflammation of the substance of the spinal cord and is similar to the two conditions above except that this condition can be caused by wounds especially impact and puncture wounds.

Signs and Symptoms

Both motor and sensory nerve tracts may be involved giving rise to a variety of symptoms such as loss of sensation in the limbs and tail or paraplegia in those animals which are severely affected. A change of gait is not uncommon. There may be a loss of control over bladder and bowel functions.

Herbal Treatment

Read what is written in this section for Encephalitis and Meningitis. If the condition is caused by a wound or impact injury consider St Johns Wort (Hypericum) internally and externally. If there is paralysis consider

Guarana as this is a nerve stimulant. Homoeopathy can be faster acting so read what is written in this section for Encephalitis and Meningitis and here and if it fits what you are seeing use it along with the herbal remedy.

Homoeopathic Treatment

Conium Mac 30C - This remedy is almost specific for animals ranging from slight ataxia to paraplegia where there is progressive upwards involvement of the disease process.

Gelsemium 30C - Mild cases showing a general weakness of the neuromuscular system may benefit from this remedy. Smaller peripheral nerves are very often affected more than the large nerve trunks e.g the nerves governing the throat and larynx.

Causticum 30C - A useful remedy for the older subject showing involvement of one particular nerve e.g the sciatic or radial giving rise to a localized paralysis. The subject may display sessile warts.

Silicea 30C - This remedy has a certain reputation in the treatment of spinal conditions and is worth considering if other symptoms agree.

Vestibular Syndrome

This condition can be common in the older dog. The severity of this disease can vary from dog to dog with some being unable to stand and others hardly effected. Many dogs recover slowly in about five days but relapses can occur sometimes a lot worse. This condition can be caused by a constricted artery or a localized infection or disease of the inner ear. Sometimes the problem is caused by a tumor pressing on a nerve. This Syndrome is sometimes referred to as a stroke but is usually damage to a nerve or the inner ear.

Signs and Symptoms

In this condition the balance area of the brain is affected with the dog showing a head tilt to the effected side, the dog may fall or circle to that side and there is a flicking movement of the eyes. There may be vomiting in the initial stages of the disease.

Herbal Treatment

Treat same as you would Epilepsy. You need to try to prescribe on the whole picture of the dog and it may be worthwhile adding Oats to the diet as this is a good nerve food or as it is properly called a Nervine Restorative. Herbs that have been used for epilepsy are Skullcap which is pretty much the specific, others to consider are Mistletoe, Gotu Kola, Hyssop, Vervain and Passion Flower. To build up the nervous system and strengthen it think of Oats, Chamomile and Valerian. The herbal actions we are mainly looking at are those of the Sedatives. If the dog is old and the condition is getting worse think of Ginkgo Biloba which will increase the blood supply to the head and maybe add to this Bacopa. One of the best herbs to consider for Vestibular Syndrome is the herb used for dizzy spells and tinnitus which is Black Cohosh, not because of its female actions as it is commonly used for but because it is a blood cleanser focused on the nervous system, I use this for 3 months as this is the blood cycle in the hope of cleaning out all the rubbish. If the condition is caused by a tumor add the herb Burdock.

Homoeopathic Treatment

Argent Nit 30C - Tendency to fall sideways and attacks of vertigo may be accompanied by vomiting, problems with eyes they are sore and red maybe weepy.

Hyoscyamus 30C - Indicated when attacks are preceded by shaking of the head and a unsteadiness of gait indicating vertigo, there may be spasmodic closing of the eyelid and the mouth is flecked with foam.

Stramonium 30C - This remedy is somewhat similar to the last one but there are usually signs before the fit such as staggering with a tendency to fall toward the left side, eyes are again dilated and staring.

Conium Mac 30C - Useful in the older animal, weakness of different kinds in the hind legs ranging from unsteady gait to a inability to rise with a progressive upwards paralysis.

Gelsemium 30C - Mild cases showing a general weakness of the neuromuscular system may benefit from this remedy. Creeping paralysis.

Tetanus (Lock Jaw)

This disease is caused by the bacterium Clostridium Tetani gaining entrance to the body through a puncture or other deep wounds that are not exposed to the air.

Signs and Symptoms - The animal walks in a unsteady manner, there is muscle stiffness and muscular spasms. Severe cases involve the central nervous system with convulsions and death from respiratory failure.

Herbal Treatment

The main herb to think of here is Hypericum also known as St Johns Wort. This herb is used as a nervine anti-viral and bacterial. Traditionally it has been used to help prevent tetanus especially in horses that have trodden on a nail that has gone through the fetlock. The treatment for horses was to pour straight tincture into the wound in the hope it would kill the bacteria. Treat all wounds with Hypericum and Calendula tinctures mixed half and half diluted with water.

Homoeopathic Treatment

The following remedies may give some relief and in mild cases may lead to cure especially if started early.

Acconitum 10M - For the fear and anxiety, always give at the first signs of a problem. Give every hour for 4 doses.

Curare 30C - Helps where muscle stiffness is prominent. Give three times daily for 7days.

Strychninum 200C - The arching of the back together with extension of limbs and head matches the symptoms of this remedy. Give twice daily for 3 days.

Hypericum 1M - This remedy may help in limiting the spread of the toxin. Give three times daily for 7 days.

Ledum 6C - This is the main remedy for puncture wounds especially if they feel cold. Give frequently in the potency.

Tetanus Nosode - Combine the nosode with the selected remedy. Use for 7 days in the 30th potency.

Wounds To Nerve Rich Areas

Some nerve rich areas are the lips, the back and especially the base of the spine. Injuries to these areas really hurt. For injuries to the nerves especially when the pain is shooting down nerve pathways for example like sciatica or to nerve rich areas especially open wounds the herb to use is St Johns Wort also known as Hypericum. In open wounds use as a lotion at about 1 to 20 or even stronger at 1 to 10 if there is a lot of pain and especially bleeding as this herb also has a astringent action which spasms the end of cut blood vessels stopping the bleeding. For external use as a lotion, this herb combines well with and complements Calendula. Homoeopaths have been using them together for hundreds of years and the combined tinctures are generally called Hypercal. Use the St Johns Wort internally in the more serious cases as it helps with the pain and can relieve anxiety. Internal Homeopathic Potencies can be just as effective. This Herb in Tincture form is a must for the first aid Kit.

Herbal Overview Of The Nervous System

One of the most important herbs in this system is Hypericum also known as St Johns Wort. This herb is anti-viral, antibacterial, anti-inflammatory, a sedative and one of our main first aid remedies for wounds which helps relieve pain and can kill the tetanus bacteria and this is only mentioning a part of its uses, always consider this when there are problems with this system especially if you don't know what the problem is. Another good herb for rebuilding this system is Oats which is a Nervine tonic also think of Valerian which is our main Tranquillizer but also a good tonic for this system. A lot of the herbs mentioned below are used in a lot of other body systems as well so when you want the action of a Nervine to use in another system try to match the herb to one used in that system as well.

Antispasmodic - Prevents or eases spasms and cramps.

Herbs - Aniseed, Angelica, Black Cohosh, Chamomile, Fennel, Horehound, Hyssop, Lime Blossom, Mistletoe, Motherwort, Rosemary, Rue, Sage, Skullcap, St johns Wort, Thyme, Valerian, Vervain.

Analgesic - Herbs that reduce pain.

Herbs - Chamomile, Dong Quai, Hops, Ladys Mantle, Passion Flower, St Johns Wort, Skullcap, Valerian, Wild Yam, Withania.

Antidepressive - Damiana, Rosemary, Skullcap ,St Johns Wort, Valerian, Vervain.

Hypnotic - This means helps you to go asleep.
Herbs - Chamomile, Hops, Passion Flower, Valerian.

Nervine - Has a beneficial effect on the nervous system, acts like a tonic to this system.

Herbs - Black Cohosh, Chamomile, Hops, Lime Blossoms, Mistletoe, Motherwort, Oats, Peppermint, Rosemary, Skullcap, St Johns Wort, Tansy, Thyme, Valerian, Vervain, Wormwood.

Sedative - Calms the nervous system and reduces stress and nervousness throughout the body.

Herbs - Black Cohosh, Chamomile, Hops, Hyssop, Motherwort, Skullcap, St Johns Wort, Valerian , Vervain.

Notes

The Urinary System

Nephritis

The acute form is probably the most common kidney conditions seen in dogs. Acute Interstitial Nephritis is usually viral or bacterial in origin with the commonest causes being infection due to the Leptospira species which is passed on by infected urine. Many Poisons such as weed killers and anti-freeze can damage the kidneys and cause similar symptoms. Another consideration to think of is has the infection traveled up the ureters from a infection further down such as cystitis or has it come via the blood from a infection elsewhere in the body.

Signs and Symptoms

These can develop quite quickly and are at first accompanied by lack of appetite and depression. The patient is thirsty and vomits a lot. A rise of temperature is seen in the early stages but may drop to near normal latter. Signs of discomfort in the lumber region are evident with tenderness over the kidney region and arching of the back. In the early stages little urine is produced but if the inflammation continues damage is done to the fine nephrons and then large quantities of dilute urine are produced. The thirst will increase when damage has been done to the nephrons. There is a disinclination to move and when the animal is encouraged to do so stiffness of movement is seen. The coat becomes dry due to dehydration while circulatory disturbance is shown by a full bounding pulse and discoloration of visible mucous membranes. Elimination of urine is decreased.

Herbal Treatment

As for any infections think of garlic, Echinacea and Myrrh and doses of Vitamin C. Try to figure the cause and fast the animal for at least a few days only giving pure honey. First lets concentrate on the inflammation with the Anti Inflammatorys here Cleavers, Golden Rod and Licorice (careful increase blood pressure) are good options as they have lots of other actions that we need as well. Other herbs good for supporting the Kidney are Bearberry and Parsley. Other actions to consider are Urinary Antiseptics and the Demulcents. So for this condition consider Bearberry , Buchu and Corn Silk which are all urinary antiseptics and two of these herbs are demulcents so they would sooth the inflamed area as well as attack the infection. Go through all the herbs at the end of the chapter listed under the Actions needed and choose the best to cover the symptoms you are seeing. Minimize Protein in the diet so as to take some work load off the kidneys.

Homoeopathic Treatment

Aconitum 12X - This should be given in the early stages, at this stage the animal shows anxiety and distress and possibly even fear. This remedy will do much to relieve the patient of these anxieties and help calm them.

Apis Mel 200C - This is a most valuable remedy especially for the edema and swelling it may also help with the pain.

Arsen Alb 1M - For animals which show dehydration and a harsh dry coat and have a thirst for small quantities of water often, the mucous membranes of the eyes are red and there may be vomiting and diarrhea. Symptoms are usually worse towards midnight when the patient becomes increasingly restless.

Belladonna 200C - The animal feels extremely hot with dilated pupils and a full bounding pulse, there are frequent attempts to pass urine which is scanty in amount and sometimes reddish brown in color. Signs of nervous system involvement may be present such as excitability and possibly a tendency to convulsions.

Phosphorus 200C - A important remedy which will help to control vomiting which arises when liquids are rejected soon after ingestion. There may be a accompanying gingivitis with small hemorrhages present when this remedy is indicated.

Urtica Urens 3X - This remedy helps elimination of waste products via the urine and promotes urination.

Chronic Nephritis

This is a progressive condition with varying degrees found in dogs over the age of 8 years old although the clinical signs may not be present in all cases. With younger animals the problem could be genetic or damage done by infections. There is no one outstanding cause and while degeneration of kidney tissue can follow the acute form it may develop by itself without any obvious symptoms.

When this condition starts pay close attention to the diet and start decreasing its protein content so as to take the work load off the kidneys. Protein breaks down to urea which the kidneys remove. Special diets can be brought for this condition.

Signs and Symptoms

As the blood urea rises the dog becomes lethargic and the appetite starts to fail. Progressive loss of weight occurs which is accompanied by stomatitis, vomiting and increased thirst. The output of urine is increased, the urine itself being pale and watery. Dehydration is a constant feature; the coat may become harsh and dry while the skin may show scattered lesions of eczema. Mouth ulcers may start and the dog may also start becoming anemic.

Herbal Treatment

You really need to know the cause to be able to give the best treatment but if in doubt you can use all the herbs mentioned in the acute condition. Remember it is the diet that is the most important as the more work we can take off what's left of the kidneys the longer they will last. For this condition I would be inclined to make up a tonic formula using the Urinary Antiseptics (Bearberry) so as to keep infections at bay along with the Demulcents so as to sooth the affected areas especially if there is pain and to this I would add Gravel Root in case a stone is causing the problem and herbs like Chaparral, Cleavers and Damiana which are Alterative to clean out the area.

Parsley is a good herb for a tonic formula.

Homoeopathic Treatment

Arsen. Alb 30C - The remedy to be considered when the patient shows excessive dehydration with increased thirst and dry coat. Itching of various areas may be pronounced and all symptoms are generally worse towards midnight, there is great restlessness.

Colchicum 30C - There is increased urination with frequency. The urine can vary from clear to dark brown. There are usually accompanying joint pains indicated by stiffness and a inclination not to move. Abdominal flatulence may be more extreme and edema may be present.

Iodum 30C - A suitable remedy for the older patient and for those animals which show wasting accompanied by a ravenous appetite. The coat is dry and superficial lymph glands may show hardness while diminishing in size. There may be frothy diarrhea of a light creamy color.

Phosphuros 30C - This remedy has a beneficial tonic effect on the kidney parenchyma. Output of urine is increased and vomiting of stomach contents when they become warm is a strong guiding symptom for its use.

Natrum Mur 30C- Excessive urination and frequency is a notable feature when this remedy may be needed and this is often worse during the night. Mouth lesions in the form of superficial ulcers and blisters are often present while hawking and scraping of throat occurs.

Cystitis

This is a frequently encountered problem that can affect dogs and especially bitches of all breeds as their urethra is shorter than a male so the infection has less distance to travel and less of the body's defenses to deal with. The cause is usually bacterial in the acute form but a significant number of cases may also be due to mechanical cases such as damage to the bladder lining due to the presence of stones which turns it into a more chronic form of disease. Strep, Staph and E Coli are the main acute causes for this problem. It is best to deal with this problem as fast as possible because the infection can travel up the ureters and infect the kidneys making a far worse condition.

Signs and Symptoms

The main sign is frequency of urination which is often attended by severe straining, the urine may be passed drop by drop and there can sometimes be blood in the urine. The animal resents pressure over the bladder region and the urine may be strong smelling and is usually dark in color.

Herbal Treatment

The main herbs we use in cystitis are the Urinary Antiseptics with the best ones being Bearberry and Buchu. Cranberry is a good urinary antiseptic too but this is used in the more chronic form of the disease as a preventative, try not to use the juice as it is not concentrated enough. To the Antiseptics we add

Demulcents which sooth and protect the irritated tissues with the best one for this condition being Corn Silk. You could add to the formula Gravel Root and Chaparral if you think the cause of the condition could be from urinary stones or gravel. Other herbs to consider are Angelica, Yarrow, Agrimony, Cleavers, Damiana, Golden Rod, Juniper, Plantain and Shepherds Purse.

Homoeopathic Treatment

Aconitum 12X - Will be of value in the early feverish phase of the acute stage, helping to calm the patient and allay pain and fear.

Cantharis 6C - One of the principle remedies employed, the patient strains violently and passes blood stained urine drop by drop with great frequency.

Causticum 30C - A useful remedy in the recurrent or chronic form and is especially adapted to the older animal. Follows well after Cantharis which may be needed if acute symptoms flare up in the chronic form.

Stone or Calculi Formation

This is a constitutional problem that has as a end result the formation of stones or gravel in the renal pelvis or bladder. Sometimes gravel can travel down one the ureters causing considerable pain. This condition is more frequent in the male dog. Stones which are mostly made up of phosphates are the most common and have their origin in alkaline urine which may predispose the dog to urinary infections as the acid helps to keep the system germ free to a certain extent. Other stones made up of cystine or urate are less common and more often happen in certain breeds caused by genetic defects. Once large stones have formed the only treatment is surgery but in the early stages there are a number of useful remedies which can prevent further deterioration and in some cases dissolve the stones. Drinking of bore water can cause stones in some animals.

Signs and Symptoms

The first signs observed are usually the passage of blood and purulent material in the urine. There may be difficulty passing urine and the urine may be very dark maybe with sediment, pain in the bladder may cause the animal to cry out or lick or gnaw at the bladder area, severe pain and discomfort attend the passage of urine which is usually voided drop by drop. If left untreated this condition leads on to kidney failure.

Herbal Treatment

The three different types of Herbal Actions we have to use here are the Urinary Antiseptics, the Demulcents (so as to sooth and protect raw areas) and the Antilithics which prevent the buildup of stones. Don't forget to use our immune boosters if infection is present they are Echinacea, Garlic and Myrrh. Also consider using Cranberry as an infection preventative as this coats the pipelines and prevents bacteria from adhering to them, they skid off and get flushed out.

Some good Urinary Antiseptics are Angelica, Bearberry and Buchu. Good demulcents for this system are Corn silk, Marshmallow and Bearberry. Some Antilithics are Cleavers, Bearberry, Gravel Root and Chaparral. Vegetables such as lovage, celery, asparagus and artichoke are good preventatives for stone formation and can be added to the diet in small quantities at first to see if they agree. Make sure the dog has lots of fresh water and drinks often. If the dog is drinking boar water stop this as it could be part of the cause. A teaspoon of apple cider vinegar in the water bowl is a good preventative for this condition.

Homoeopathic Treatment

Calc Phos 30C - A good constitutional remedy which will help regulate the calcium and phosphate metabolism and so prevent the formation of phosphates. it should be given as a routine remedy in young animals up till the age of one.

Lycopodium 30C - This remedy has a tonic action on the liver and will help to control the metabolism of that gland as a disturbed liver is frequently the cause of gravel formation. Subjects are thin and wizened looking showing reddish sediment in the urine.

Mag Mur 6C - May help in preventing some forms of stones and may be given as a routine remedy if the urine shows suspicious deposits and there are other signs of stone formation.

Urtica Urens 3X - Thickens the urine and removes the tendency to gravel formation by removing the basic salts that help form it, it will also increase the quantity of urine passed.

Prostatitis

This condition is fairly uncommon in dogs and can be seen at any age. Acute inflammation of the gland can arise independently of any enlargement and is usually due to a bacterial infection giving symptoms of elevated temperature and pulse. Vets normally take a culture and try to match a anti biotic to it.

Signs and Symptoms

The dog is subdued and off its food and usually has a temperature. The animal usually adopts a posture with the back arched which appears to give relief from the pain and may be reluctant to move. The dog may strain to pass urine which may have traces of blood.

Herbal Treatment

If the inflammation is caused from infection then we must think of our immune boosters Echinacea, Garlic and Myrrh. Our main herbs will be the Urinary Antiseptics Angelica, Bearberry, Buchu and Corn Silk. Bearberry and Corn Silk have a Demulcent action which make them a handy herb as they do two jobs at once but another good one to add would be Marshmallow. Other herbs to consider are those mentioned in the Enlarged Prostrate section. Also look at the Anti-Inflammatory herbs and for this condition concentrate on treating the pain.

Homoeopathic treatment

Aconitum 30C - To be considered in all early stages

where its use will relieve anxiety and help to calm the animal.

Belladonna 30C - If the symptoms of dilated pupils, throbbing pulse and body heat are present this will be the remedy.

Hepar Sulph 200C - In this strength the remedy will help allay the tendency to abscess formation.

Sabal 6C - Enlarged prostate, constant desire to pass water at night.

Soldago 30C - A good remedy for when there are unsuccessful attempts at urination

Enlarged Prostate Gland

This condition is fairly common in the older dog with still functioning testicles. The enlarged gland may contain cysts which give it a nodular feel. These also give the urine a discolored appearance due to the presence of cystic fluid. The enlarged prostrate can also press upon the bowel and cause faecal straining or constipation. Vets sometimes treat this condition by giving large doses of female hormones.

Signs and Symptoms

There may be straining on passing urine or moving the bowels. Diagnosis is by rectal examination or x-ray.

Herbal Treatment

Herbs that are used for the treatment of the prostrate in order of importance are Saw Palmetto, Epilobium, Horsetail, Parsley and Corn Silk, add to these any other herbs that are used in the urinary system to cover other symptoms with the condition so your formula is as wholistic as possible. If there is trouble with constipation change the diet to one with more fiber.

Homoeopathic Treatment

Apis Mel 30C - Helps to reduce cystic fluid
Sabal 6C - Enlarged prostate, constant desire to pass water at night.
Soldago 30C - A good remedy for when there are unsuccessful attempts at urination

Herbal Overview Of The Urinary System

Most infections get to the kidneys via the blood for the kidneys are the main filter of the blood removing wastes and water. Other infections can start off as cystitis and travel up the ureter and infect the kidney that way so you must always consider both ways. Always ask yourself is the infection traveling from the kidney down or the bladder up? If you think it is the kidney put a leash on the animal and walk them in tight circles one way and then the other. If the animal complains it is probably the kidney. Urinary antiseptics are good for this system whether for treating infection or preventing it as in cases of stones scraping the sides as they go down leaving a wound ripe for infection. Also think of Cranberry for this system as it coats the pipes and stops bacteria getting a foot hold literally.

Herbal Actions For The Urinary System

Anti-biotic - Chaparral, Echinacea, Garlic, Myrrh, Pau D' Arco.

Anti-inflammatory - Helps the body to combat inflammations.

Herbs - Cats Claw, Chaparral , Cleavers, Cranesbill, Eyebright, Ginger, Golden Rod, Guaiacum, Licorice, Marshmallow, Pau D' Arco.

Anti-lithic - Prevent the formation of stones or gravel in the urinary system and helps the body to remove them.

Herbs - Bearberry, Corn Silk, Chaparral, Gravel Root, Horsetail.

Anti-microbial - Helps the body destroy or resist pathogenic micro-organisms.

Herbs - Echinacea, Garlic, Juniper, Myrrh,

Astringent - Contracts tissue which in turn reduces discharges, these herbs contain tannins.

Herbs - Agrimony, Cranesbill, Chaparral, Golden Rod, Horsetail, Shepherds Purse.

Cystitis - Agrimony, Bearberry, Buchu, Celery Seed, Corn Silk, Gravel Root, Golden Rod, Horsetail, Plantain,

Demulcent - Soothes and protects irritated or inflamed internal tissues.

Herbs - Bearberry, Corn Silk, Licorice, Marshmallow, Plantain, Slippery Elm.

Diuretic - Increases the secretion and elimination of urine. Generally has a action on the kidneys.

Herbs - Agrimony Angelica, Bear Berry, Blue Flag, Burdock, Buchu, Broom, Coltsfoot, Chaparral, Corn Silk, Dandelion Leaves, Elder, Fumitory, Golden Rod, Guaiacum, Gravel Root, Hawthorn, Horseradish, Horsetail, Juniper, Lime Blossom, Nettles, Pau D' Arco, Penny Royal, Plantain, Parsley, Shepherds Purse, Sarsaparilla, Yarrow.

Urinary Antiseptics - These herbs have a antiseptic action as they pass through the system.

Herbs - Angelica, Bearberry, Buchu, Corn Silk, Golden Rod, Shepherds Purse, Yarrow.

Notes

The Musculo-Skeletal System

Osteoporosis

A condition in which bones become increasingly porous. It is due to metabolic upsets and may follow a systemic disease. Diagnosis depends on X -ray but symptoms can be a increased tendency to fractures. One cause is an all meat diet so check out nutrition.

Herbal Treatment

This really depends on what is the cause of the problem is it nutrition, assimilation or is it a metabolic type of problem caused by a problem with the liver. I think here it is best to find the cause before using herbs. Generally the cause of the problem is diet and age.

Homoeopathic Treatment

Calc Phos 30C - This is a very useful remedy for the younger animal in the growing stage as it exerts a profound influence on the development of bone and muscle. More suitable for lean animals.

Calc Carb 30C - This remedy has a action similar to the above one but it suits the fat animal more than the lean one.

Silicea 30C - This is a good tissue remedy exerting a beneficial action on the skeleton in general.

Osteomyelitis

This term refers to a infection of the bone in the acute form which arises when bacteria gains entrance to the medulla of the bone either through blood transfer or via compound fractures.

Chronic osteomyelitis can develop when infections reach the periosteum (covering of the bone) and can follow puncture wounds and bites. In the foot access can be gained by a damaged nail bed. Bone infections are normally localized to the area. The main organisms associated with this disease are Staphylococci and to a lesser extent Streptococci.

Signs and Symptoms

Acute disease is characterized by lameness, heat and swelling of the limb along with pain. Sinus formation with purulent discharge is often the early sign of the chronic form along with the dog going off their food and maybe becoming lethargic with sometimes a raised temperature. In severe cases the infection can weaken the bone so much that it may fracture. X-ray is a good way for diagnosis.

Herbal Treatment

For this condition think of our infection fighting herbs such as Echinacea, Garlic and Myrrh. If the skin is broken and you think the infection got in this way apply a lotion of Calendula and Hypericum to the area and keep doing so until the wound is closed. Treat the symptoms as you see them, if there is inflammation use the Anti Inflammatorys. Alteratives may be needed as well so as to clean out the area and system; some examples of herbs that have both of these actions are Devils Claw and Sarsaparilla. Think of Comfrey in the latter stages of healing but never use at the beginning of a condition such as this as it seals the wound to fast.

Homoeopathic Treatment

Aconitum 30C - Should always be given in the early febrile stage and may have to be repeated for one or two doses.

Hepar Sulph 30C - In the acute form accompanying severe pain this could prove a very useful remedy. A guiding symptom for its use is extremely sensitive to pain.

Ruta 6C - This remedy has a beneficial action on infections or inflammations of the periosteum and should be of good use in the acute form and may prevent the chronic from arising.

Calc Phos 30C and Calc Carb 30C - These two remedies could prove useful in treatment of the young animal that is still developing.

Silica 30C - A suitable remedy for the chronic form where sinuses have formed.

Symphytum 200C - This remedy should help allay the tendency to any weakening of bone structure and is generally a good healing agent.

Myositis

Inflammation of muscle fibers leading to degeneration in prolonged cases. The cause may be systemic (Bacterial infection) or traumatic (injury).

Signs and Symptoms

There may be swelling of the muscle involved but frequently no signs are evident except for the fact that the animal cries out on being moved or lifted. Various postures are assumed according to the muscles affected eg the arching of the back when the lumber muscles are affected or maybe a board like feeling on the abdomen which indicates pain of the muscles at that region.

Herbal Treatment

If the cause is from bacterial infection then we would use our immune boosting herbs so as to start fighting the infection, these are Echinacea, Myrrh and Garlic. If inflammation is present treat with Anti-Inflammatories especially the ones that are pain killers - Willow bark and Devils Claw. If the inflammation was caused by injury try some of the First Aid remedies such as a compress of Arnica Lotion. Don't forget to look at the Homoeopathic First Aid remedies.

Homoeopathic Treatment

Aconitum 6C - Should always be considered in the early stages and will bring about relief from pain especially if the origin is bacterial. It will allay any tendency to shock if the condition arises quickly.

Rhus Tox 6C - Indicated when the animal gains relief from movement even though the initial movement is painful, symptoms may be more on the left side of the body then the right, indicated when severe wetting or prolong dampness is associated with the onset of the symptoms.

Bryonia 30C - Movement is resented when Bryonia is indicated. The animal will seek to lie on the affected muscles and pressure on them gives ease, warmth is usually useful also.

Causticum 30C - This remedy is associated with a accompanying contraction of tendons and a stiffness of muscles, warmth gives relief, more adaptable to the older patient with unsteadiness of gait.

Gelsemium 30C - Weakness and a tendency to paralysis is the keynote of this remedy. There may be generalized involvement of all muscles and the trouble is usually systemic in origin, an attempt to exercise the animal can lead to collapse and severe fatigue.

Osteoarthritis

Degenerative joint disease where the articular cartilages become eroded and bony exostoses occur at the margin of the joints. The hip and stifle joints are the ones most commonly affected. Osteoarthritis is mainly caused by wear and tear and as a result of old injuries.

All though age plays a part there can be other causes such as systemic or metabolic disturbances or a all protein diet which makes too much acid for the body to deal with. Progressive mild inflammation in the joint over a period of time is more likely to produce osteoarthritis than any other predisposing factor. Osteoarthritis particularly affects the load bearing bones of the body. Being overweight adds to the wear and tear of the joints. Once the cartilage degenerates the cushioning effect is lost within the joint and the joint capsule now becomes involved and the situation becomes worse.

Signs and Symptoms

Lameness is the main sign and it could involve several joints. A unwillingness to use the affected part results in muscular wasting of the area, later signs include thickening of the joint, the worst affected limb may be held in a flexed manner.

Herbal Treatment

Nutrition wise for the early stages you can give calcium, Vitamin D, magnesium and manganese so as to try to stop the condition from getting worse and ensure the animal is getting a balanced diet with not too much protein. Glucosamine and Chondroitin Sulphate can help stimulate the rebuilding of cartilage and help in the early stages of arthritis and prevent other parts of the body from becoming affected.

Arthritis with lots of pain and inflammation needs the use of the Anti-Inflammatory herbs, good ones to use for this condition are Meadowsweet, Devils Claw and Willow bark as these act as good pain killers as well. Other herbs to use are the Alteratives which clean out the area and the system some good ones are Burdock, Garlic, Sarsaparilla and Chaparral which has a antioxidant action as well. Diuretic herbs are also used for this condition as they help to remove the metabolic waste and toxins which usually result from the constant inflammation and help the kidneys flush this waste out, some good ones are Celery Seed, Juniper (these two are best used together) and

Dandelion leaf. Other herbs to look at for arthritis are Black Cohosh, Cats Claw, Guaiacum, Nettles, Wild yam and Yellow dock. Add Licorice to the formula at about 10% as this will help in the assimilation of the formula into the body. Excess acid has a lot to do with this condition so for this consider Celery Seed which is known as the acid remover and also Meadowsweet which is known as the Acid Balancer.

Homoeopathic Treatment

Bryonia 6C - The animal prefers to remain still and any movement causes distress and sometimes acute pain evidenced by the animal crying out.

Caulophyllum 6C - This remedy could be indicated if the condition is confined to the smaller joints eg, carpus, tarsus and the joints of the toes.

Calc Flour 30C - may be needed in the latter stages once the exostoses and joint swellings develop. The carpus is the main joint affected when this remedy is indicated. There may be accompanying cystic tumors around the joint.

Rhus Tox 6C - This remedy is indicated when the animal's symptoms are eased after a short period of movement, there may be initial stiffness on first moving.

Arthritis due to Infection

This is caused by pyogenic bacteria getting in the joint mainly from injury the main organisms are Streptococci and Staphylococci .

Signs and Symptoms

There is an initial temperature rise and febrile (heat) signs develop. The affected joint becomes swollen, tense and hot. Pain is obvious by the onset of severe lameness. Examination may reveal the presence of punctures on the skin and the appearance of a purulent exudate.

Herbal Treatment

For this condition think of our infection fighting herbs such as Echinacea, Garlic and Myrrh. If the skin is broken and you think the infection got in this way apply a lotion of Calendula and Hypericum to the area. To our infection fighting herbs you can add some of the Anti Inflammatories, Alteratives and Diuretics that are mentioned in Osteoarthritis but mainly here concentrate on the infection. Add Licorice to the formula at about 10% as this will help in the assimilation of the formula into the body and help as a good anti-inflammatory.

Homoeopathic Treatment

Aconitum 30C - This should be given as soon as possible in the early febrile stage.

Apis Mel 6C - If the synovial sheaf of the joint becomes edematous indicated by swelling this remedy may help. The patient is made worse by heat in any form and does not drink much.

Belladonna 30C - Indicated when the patient presents a excitable picture with dilated pupils, throbbing arteries and a hot skin.

Bryonia 6C - Symptoms worse for movement, relief

from pain on pressure over the joint and a possible involvement with the respiratory tract. The joint is usually extremely hard and tense.

Ferrum Phos 6C - This also is a good remedy for the initial feverish stage more often indicate when throat symptoms accompany the invasive process.

Ledum 6C - The remedy of choice if the arthritis has been caused by the penetration of a sharp object giving rise to a puncture wound.

Iodum 6C - This is a remedy which sometimes gives good results in the less acute case especially when the joint pains are worse at night. The patient is often thin with a voracious appetite and the skin is dry and withered looking.

Rhus Tox 6C - The indications for this remedy are relief from movement although there may be initial stiffness on rising. There may be accompanying skin symptoms of a vesicular itchy nature.

Silica 30C - This remedy is indicated in the more chronic case. There may be involvement of neighboring lymphatic glands showing cold abscesses.

Bursitis

By this term we mean the appearance of a swelling over the joint, those commonly affected being the points of the elbows and the hock. Damage to the bursa of the joint due to overweight is a common contributory factor as is also irritation of the part by repeated contact with the ground if the animal is inclined to rest more than usual.

Signs and Symptoms

The acute form shows swelling, heat and pain evidenced by lameness. Effusion into the bursa occurs and accounts in part to the increase of size. When bursitis is chronic changes take place leading to the formation of a solid lump in the affected area. This may eventually ulcerate leading to secondary infection.

Herbal Treatment

Liniments made from essential oils in a base of olive oil can be applied to the area, Cayenne and Ginger would increase the circulation to the area while Wintergreen would act as a good pain killer along with Peppermint. Other essential oils are St Johns Wort, Lavender and Rosemary.

If the condition is becoming chronic or even if it seems painful treat with the herbs mentioned under Anti-Inflammatorys but still also apply oils directly to the area.

Homoeopathic Treatment

Apis Mel 30C - Useful in the early inflammatory stage where effusion is taking place and the joint is extremely tender to touch, the animal may lick and gnaw at the joint because of itching and irritation. Patient shows a intolerance to heat and touch. Apis is always good for sharp pains and swellings.

Bryonia 6C - Indicated when the joint is enlarged and pressure over the area brings relief as does the application of cold compresses. The animal resents movement and prefers to lie on the effected joint.

Rhus Tox 6C - If surrounding ligaments and tendons are involved to any great extent this remedy will be needed, movement limbers up the animal which is in need of Rhus Tox.

Calc Flour 30C - This is a good general tissue remedy and has a beneficial effect on the development of cysts, cystic tumors and fibrous swellings.

Silica 30C - This is another good long term remedy which will help dissolve any associated scar and fibrous tissue. It will be beneficial if surface ulceration occurs leading to secondary infection.

Bone Injuries and Fractures

Herbal Treatment

The main remedy here is Comfrey or to use its old fashioned name knitbone. This is good to use internally and on the injured area when the cast is removed as it will help to strengthen the mend. For areas that do not have casts on or for fine fractures Comfrey is ideal and will speed up the healing process. Comfrey has a chemical in it that speeds up cell division it is also Astringent and Demulcent which gives it soothing and protecting qualities and has been used for hundreds of years in the healing of bones and wounds. Some people grow this herb and then turn it into liquid manure as it is one of the most mineral rich herbs around.

Treatment

Apply cream to affected area regularly, if you grow

Comfrey in your garden you can make a poultice out of the leaves and apply it to the affected area.

Homoeopathic Treatment

Follow normal first aid procedures, if the bone is obviously broken it is best to call a vet. If you do have to move the patient make sure the injured limb is supported or a sharp piece of bone may cut a internal artery. Plastic plumbing pipe split down the middle makes a excellent splint. Most bone injuries need x-rays to determine the extent of the damage.

Remedies with leading symptoms

Arnica 6 to 30C - Can be given straight away for the shock and will help ease the pain from the bruising and swelling.

Ledum 6 to 30C - Take after arnica 4 hourly or 3 times a day to assist in the absorption of the extravasation of blood after a fracture so as to reduce the swelling which may take up to 3 to 4 days. (Helps to absorb the internal bleeding after a fracture)

After the bones have been set properly use these two remedies.

Calc Phos 6X - Helps in nutrition especially of the bones and promotes the knitting together of the bones. Helps fractures heal much faster. Can be used in alternation with Symphytum. Calc Phos is what is known as a Biochemic Tissue Salt and can be brought in most chemists.

Symphytum 6 to 30C - More commonly known as Comfrey or knitbone or bone set. The name says it all. Promotes fast healing of bones, use with Calc Phos

6X. Take both 3 times daily till recovered.

Sprains and Strains

Herbal Treatment

Severe sprains usually need a supporting bandage and a medical checkup to see if there has been any other damage. A lot of damage and trauma can be prevented if the injured area was put under cold water or ice immediately after the injury the quicker the less the damage. For a bad sprain I would use lots of Arnica cream to start with and at night apply Arnica and Comfrey mixed creams along with a support bandage for the area so as to keep the cream there and also for the extra heat to the area that would create. If you grow Comfrey in your garden then you could put on a Comfrey poultice at night. Ginger is another herb that could be used in a poultice at night.

Treatment

Cold water or ice immediately

Arnica Cream (do not apply on open wounds)

Comfrey Cream mixed with arnica cream overnight

Ginger poultice overnight.

Comfrey poultice overnight.

Calendula - Healing and soothing.

Homoeopathic Treatment

Joint problems due to twisting, wrenching or over use. A sprain is damaged tendons or ligaments while a strain happens when the connecting tissues around a joint are over stretched. Use your normal first aid procedures and support the joint with supporting bandage and give the appropriate remedies with the first one being Arnica. If there is no sign of improvement in 24 to 36 hours get checked for a fracture.

Arnica 6 to 30C - For the shock and bruised sore pains. Arnica cream can also be applied as long as the skin is not broken.

Bellis Perennis 6 to 30C - Deeper acting then arnica, intense soreness of the muscles, where swellings and lumps remain after the injury.

Ledum 6 to 30C - Injuries where the swollen part is cold or numb, sometimes looks purple and puffy, feels better for cold applications.

Ruta 6 to 30C - If the bones inside or near the joint feel bruised

Herbal Overview Of The Muscular Skeletal System

For bruising think about Arnica in a lotion and use the Homoeopathic dose internally, for broken bones think about Comfrey as its old name is knit bone. For arthritis and rheumatism use your Anti Rheumatics, Anti Inflammatorys, and Analgesics but also think of Celery Seed as this is called the acid remover and another herb to think of is Meadowsweet as this herb is called the acid balancer. It is usually the high acid in the system that irritates the joints and starts the inflammation so these 2 herbs could remove the cause for the condition, also consider diet as a diet high in protein will create a lot of acid waste. For blood borne bacterial infections think of the Alteratives (blood cleansers) and Anti Bacterials especially our main ones Garlic and Echinacea. If there is damage to the joints use a nutritional supplement with these 3 together - Glucosamine Sulphate, Chondroitin and MSM as these together will help rebuild the joints.

Herbal Actions For The Muscular Skeletal System

Alterative - Herbs that gradually restore proper function to the body, they increase health and vitality. They were once known as the blood cleansers.

Herbs - Black Cohosh, Blue Flag, Burdock, Chaparral, Echinacea, Garlic, Nettles, Pau D'Arco ,Sarsaparilla, Yellow Dock.

Analgesic - Herbs that reduce pain.

Herbs - Black Cohosh, Chamomile, Hops, Meadowsweet, Pau D'Arco, Peppermint, Skullcap, St Johns Wort, Valerian.

Anti-biotic - Chaparral, Echinacea, Garlic, Myrrh, Pau D' Arco.

Antispasmodic - Prevents or eases spasms and cramps.

Herbs - Angelica, Black Cohosh, Chamomile, Skullcap, St johns Wort, Valerian.

Anti-inflammatory - Helps the body to combat inflammations.

Herbs - Cats Claw, Devils Claw, Chaparral , Feverfew, Ginger, Guaiacum, Liquorice,

Meadowsweet, Pau D' Arco, Sarsaparilla, St Johns Wort, Willow Bark.

Anti-viral - Astragalus, Cats claw, Echinacea, Garlic, Myrrh?, St Johns Wort, Pau D'Arco.

Anti-Rheumatic - Angelica, Burdock, Black Cohosh, Chaparral, Cats Claw, Celery Seed, Dandelion, Garlic, Guaiacum, Nettles, Willow Bark, Yellow Dock.

Rubefacient - Causes a gentle local irritation to the skin which stimulates the capillaries to open increasing the blood flow.

Herbs - Cayenne, Garlic, Ginger, Horseradish, Nettles, Peppermint Oil, Rosemary Oil, Rue.

Notes

Diseases of the Skin

Allergic Skin Diseases

These occur frequently in a form that looks like dermatitis, they are often encountered in the summer though they can turn chronic and be all year round. Skin allergies can be caused by external and internal causes. Dogs can be allergic to many things some are pollens, grasses, fleas and other insects, foods, detergents and materials just to list a few. Here we really need to find the cause, is it seasonal, is it all the time in which case it could be food or something in the environment that the dog comes into contact with. If you think it is environment send the dog to a friend's place for a week and see what happens, if you think it is diet change this to a more natural diet and see what happens.

Signs and Symptoms

Generalized itching is present in most cases and may be more severe when the skin becomes exposed to warmth or becomes aggravated by cold conditions. The skin itself may show slight to moderate redness without any other changes or become thickened and be accompanied by a degree of baldness. The abdomen and inner thighs particularly show an redness and maybe a papular rash.

In flea bite allergies over the back and in front of the tail will be the most affected area. Eczemas of various types can be considered under this heading although not all forms of eczema are allergic in origin. They may be acute or chronic, wet or dry with clinical signs and symptoms similar to those outlined above. Severe itching may cause secondary infections from scratching.

Herbal Treatment

Remove the cause is about the best treatment you can give if it is known. Albizzia is known as a anti-allergy herb and is the main one to try along with Vitamin C for this vitamin is a strong Anti-histamine. Another herb to consider is Garlic because this is also Antihistamine and its Antibacterial Action will help to prevent infection of over scratched areas. I would also be inclined to give the Alterative herbs so as to clean out the system as toxic systems can cause allergy problems. Good ones to use are Burdock, Cleavers, Chaparral, Fumitory, Goto kola and Sarsaparilla just to mention a few. Herbs you could apply to the skin in a lotion or cream are Chickweed whose main leading symptom is itching, Calendula which is anti-inflammatory, healing and soothing as well as germicide (these two herbs together would be a good combination) and another herb to try is Neem which is more focused to the flea and parasite killing side (has a effect on their reproductive systems) as well as having a action on the skin.

Homoeopathic Treatment

Sulphur 30 or 200C - Indicated when the skin is red and itching is intense, made worse by heat. The gums may be unduly red. Papular or vesicular rash may also be present to. It is a good undercurrent remedy and may be given with other remedies to enhance their action or at the beginning of treatment generally.

Arsen Alb 30C to 1M - When the skin is dry and scaly, shedding of epidermal cells occurring and accompanied by harsh, lusterless hair. The animal seeks warmth and shows a desire for small quantities of water taken frequently. Symptoms become worse after midnight and other systemic disturbances may include diarrhea of cadaverous odor.

Rhus Tox 6C to 1M - This remedy should be considered when the skin symptoms are aggravated by wet and the dog shows stiffness when moving after rest but moves more easily when exercise proceeds. The skin shows papular or vesicular rash with much itching and redness. Warmth lessens the severity of the symptoms.

Antimonium Crud 6C - When skin lesions are more pronounced on the neck, back and limbs taking the form of papular eruptions which latter become scabby discharging a yellowish secretion. Itching is worse towards evening and aggravated by warmth.

Hepar Sulph 200c - The remedy of choice when lesions show extreme sensitivity to external stimuli and pus is beginning to form. The skin is usually swollen and shiny with a tense appearance. It is helpful in drying up the underlying purulent discharge in those cases with crusts and scabs.

Acute Bacterial Dermatitis

Various organisms may be implicated but the commonest are Staphylococcal and Streptococcal frequently producing a mixed infection. Treat Folliculitis and Impetigo the same way as mentioned below for they are all bacterial skin conditions.

Signs and Symptoms

The initial lesion takes the form of a rash, the vesicles form a raw area which exudes serum. Severe irritation is set up causing the animal to lick the area more or less constantly enlarging the original lesions. Purulent material is soon evident because of secondary infection.

Herbal Treatment

Treat internally with immune system boosters like Echinacea, Myrrh and Garlic, maybe add some Alteratives from the herbal section below especially if the condition has been going on for a while. The original lesion should never have been allowed to get as bad as described in the symptoms it should of been treated with a lotion of Calendula immediately. If the dog is gnawing on the wound and it is a fairly bad wound cover it in a gauze bandage and soak the bandage with a lotion of Calendula keeping the dressing wet. Consider mixing Chickweed with the Calendula if you think itching is part of the problem. The dog could be fitted with a Elizabethan collar and sent to rest a few days in the barn. Look at the section on wounds.

Homoeopathic Treatment

The affected areas should be washed clean with a warm lotion containing Calendula and Hypericum lotion at a strength of 1 to 10 also consider the Chick

Weed mentioned above if the dog is constantly scratching, then choose from the following remedies.

Sulphur 6C or 30C - This remedy should always be given first as it helps clear the blood of impurities which could add to the general inflammatory state. This is a good remedy for itching.

Rhus Tox 1M - Useful for the initial vesicular stage with redness and swelling. Severe itching is present causing the vesicles to rupture and produce a red area. Scratching does not relieve.

There may be associated symptoms suggesting rheumatism such as difficulty in rising but symptoms are generally improved by movement. The animal is very restless.

Antimonum Crud 6C - When this remedy is indicated lesions are seen more often on the upper parts of the body and are worse in the evening. The vesicles have a nettle rash appearance and may appear like measles discharging a blood stained exudate. Itching is intense and symptoms are worse by warmth and from touch. Signs of alimentary disturbances may be seen such as disinclination to eat and vomiting.

Mange

The most severe variety of mange is canine Scabies. Sarcoptic Mange is caused by the mite Sarcoptes scabiei, which also causes human scabies. The mite burrows into the skin to lay eggs and what happens then is serum, the clear component of the blood, seeps out of the tunnels to the surface of the skin and causes thick scabs to form.

Animals must be isolated as this is a very infectious condition which can be passed on to humans. Survival of the mite egg away from the host is limited. The mite parasite feeds on the host but can live for up to 21 days without feeding. Mites can therefore be found anywhere in the environment and special attention must be paid to ensuring brushes, combs, collars, bedding, carpeting and all upholstered surfaces are sprayed with an insecticide.

Signs and Symptoms - The main symptoms are Frantic Itching and scratching which can open the skin to infection. In severe cases the skin becomes thickened, pigmented and scurfy. Other signs are loss of hair with the first stages usually affecting patches around the ears, elbows, legs, and face, with later stages having patches around the whole body. Crusting of the skin forms along with scab formation. The hair loss is characterized by patches of approximately one inch in diameter. Dogs with scabies may often dig and bite at themselves with great ferocity.

Herbal Treatment

Herbs used externally for this condition are Garlic, Rue, Wormwood, and Neem. A small portion of ammonia can be added to the external preparations or you could add 50% vinegar. Lemon juice has also traditionally been used for mange. A couple of bulbs of garlic could be put into the blender with a little water then blended and painted onto the affected areas. Dose the animal internally with Garlic and Wormwood with Garlic at about 70%. For this condition Pat Coleby makes up a wash of a tablespoon of Copper Sulfate and a tablespoon of cider vinegar in 500mls of water and paints this on 3 times a day, she also says look at correcting the diet.

Mange Treatment Blend With Essential Oils

15ml base oil of hazel nut or sweet almond oil

5 drops Lavender

7 drops Niaouli

1 drop Helichrysum

2 drops Sweet Marjoram

After bathing the dog 2 to 4 drops of the blend should be applied to the affected areas twice a day for at least 2 weeks. Observe for a week and repeat if necessary. Try to prevent the dog from licking the area.

Homoeopathic Treatment

Sulphur 30C - Lesions are red and look wet, itching is intense, worse for warmth. Dose night and morning for 5 days.

Arsenic Alb 30C - If the hair falls off and the skin becomes loose and flabby or if there are ulcers with hard red edges, dry eczema, animal is thirsty and seeks warmth, symptoms worse after midnight, animal becomes more restless. This remedy is good to alternate with Sulphur. Dose once daily for 2 weeks.

Sepia 30C - If the effected parts are tender and the animal shrinks when touched or if there are white looking blisters filled with a watery fluid. Dose 3 times a day.

Rhus Tox 30C- Condition is vesicular and itchy, stiffness in joints which gets better with movement. Dose 3 times daily.

Bruises

Bruises are usually impact injuries caused by blows or falls and usually heal fairly fast. When there has been substantial bruising or a high enough impact to cause shock consider using the remedies below. Bruises are caused from blood vessels that have ruptured under the skin as a result of trauma, as the blood from the broken vessels is slowly absorbed the color slowly disappears.

Herbal Treatment

Arnica is the main remedy that is used for bruising mainly as a lotion or a cream but it must not be used where the skin is broken. If used on broken skin it will cause a bad reaction. Arnica is good for the bruised like pain in limbs and joints which have been over used or sprained as well as your everyday type of bruises. Cold compresses can bring relief as well.

For bruises where there are open wounds such as cuts and grazes use St Johns Wort and Calendula together in a lotion and later you could mix the creams together and apply as healing resumes.

Homoeopathic Treatment

Arnica 6 to 30C - For bruised soft tissues, muscles and connective tissue. Rapidly aids in the absorption of effused blood. The swelling which usually accompanies bruising reduces fairly quickly but if there is little reaction use **Ledum**. Arnica cream can be used on the external area of the wound.

Caution - Arnica must not be used on or near broken skin only use Calendula or Hypericm cream on wounds.

Bellis Perennis 6 to 30C - Follows after and is similar to arnica but is used for the deeper internal bruising while arnica is more external. Good for trauma and wounds of the pelvic and abdominal organs.

Ledum 6 to 30C - Helps in blood reabsorbing, may be needed if swelling remains after taking arnica. Affected parts are cold and worse for warmth.

Hypericum 6 to 30C - For bruised nerves, use where there is sharp shooting pains in punctured or penetrating wounds, for bruises of nerve rich areas such as the fingers, tail bone, lips and nose. Hypercal cream can be applied to the site externally.

Ruta 6 to 30C - Bruises of the bone or the bone covering the periosteum, good for shin bone injuries.

Note - Hypercal cream can be used externally on bruises where the skin is broken as arnica cream or lotion cannot be used on broken skin.

Abscesses and Boils

These are typically caused by a bacterial infection usually starting in a hair follicle but anything that irritates the skin can cause a abscess. The first stage is characterized by a painful red swelling after which pus begins to form, this will usually discharge itself in a few days. Do not squeeze as this usually causes internal damage and a spread of the wound and infection.

Signs and Symptoms - The area will be swollen, red and painful to touch. Dogs tend to get them more around the head and neck

Herbal Treatment

For lots of boils or recurring boils think of a course of Echinacea and Garlic maybe followed by Burdock so as to clean up the blood especially think of this when they come in crops. Hot poultices are very effective at drawing the core out of boils so here we shall use a hot poultice of Slippery Elm (half a tea spoon full) with about 4 drops of Castor Oil which is also good at drawing out unwanted matter, mix this with a bit of boiling water to form a hot paste. Apply to the area and leave on for 20 minutes and repeat several times till suppuration occurs. After suppuration you can mix together a bit of Calendula and Comfrey creams and apply them to the area. These two herbs working together will speed up the healing time, disinfect and reduce or prevent scaring. Tea Tree Oil is also good for drawing boils and keeping the surrounding area bacteria free.

Homoeopathic Treatment

A boil is a infected, reddened, swollen area of the skin usually in a hair follicle or some other pit in the skin. Boils can be very painful while they develop until they come to a head and burst.

Remedies with leading symptoms

Hypericum Lotion - Make at a strength of 1 to 25 parts water ,soak a compress and apply reasonably wet to the affected area. Take Tarantula at the time.

Hepar Sulph 6C - To ripen a slow forming boil or abscess.

Silica 6C- For more advanced boils to encourage them to discharge, for foul smelling discharges or incomplete discharges.

Tarantula cubenis 6C - For painful hard feeling boils that develop rapidly after a slow start especially on the back of the neck or on boils where the skin turns red blue or purple. Give this remedy 3 or 4 times daily along with a Hypericum compress taped over the area.

Burns

If you live in countries like Australia then fire is common and you will have to deal with it at least once in your life. Get all burns under cold water immediately; always remember that burns keep on burning inwards for about 15 seconds after the heat source is removed. On first degree burns the skin becomes red only. 2nd degree the burn begins to destroy living tissue, blisters develop, 3rd degree the burns are deep and involve all layers of the skin, these are life threatening depending on the size of the area mainly through the loss of fluids and the risk of infections.

Herbal Treatment

For minor burns and scolds Aloe Vera gel straight from the plants leaf can give quick relief and speed up the healing. In herbal medicine we use the Astringents for burns (with the exception being for burns that cover a very large area) as the tannins in the herbs will seal and protect the burned surface and they also have a antibiotic action. Deep burns always require prompt medical attention. As the burns begin to heal you can use a mixture of Calendula and St Johns Wort cream on the healing edges.

Aloe Vera - Apply to burn straight from the plant.

Witch Hazel - Use as a lotion at about 1 to 20 strength and apply to the burn, this herb is a strong astringent and should seal and protect the surface.

Once the healing has begun you can continue applying Aloe vera especially if there is still pain. Another good herb for the pain is St Johns Wort which you could apply as a lotion. The best way to do this is from a spray bottle that gives off a fine mist.

Homoeopathic Treatment

Remedies with leading symptoms.

Calendula Cream - Use this on the edges of the burn as the burn heals.

Causticum 6 to 30C - For 2nd degree burns taken as needed for the pain with Hypericum lotion used externally on the burn and calendula cream on the edges.

Cantharis 6 to 30C - For 3rd degree burns taken as needed. This time wait for the healing to begin before using Hypericum and calendula as mentioned with Causticum.

Hypericum - To be used as a lotion 20 drops of tincture to 1 cup of water. (soothes the pain).

Urtica Urens 6 to 30C - For first degree burns taken as needed internally for the pain with Hypericum lotion used externally.

Cuts and Wounds
Herbal Treatment
The first consideration is to stop the bleeding, rule out any deeper internal damage and clean and disinfect the wound. To stop the bleeding use astringents and pressure. Calendula is one of the main lotions used for cleaning wounds as it is gentle, soothing, healing and anti-microbial so it kills the germs as well. Calendula has a tendency of sometimes welding the skin together (handy for closing knife like cuts) this is more noticeable on wounds with clean cut edges. Because of this tendency it is very important to make sure that all wounds are very clean and no dirt remains inside. I use Hypericum (St Johns Wort) lotion on wounds that are in very nerve rich areas, a good example is crush injuries to the lips as we all know how painful and sensitive a wound is to this area. As well as being used for nerve damage Hypericm is also astringent so it will help in stopping the bleeding and its anti-inflammatory action should help to reduce the swelling, this herb is also used to prevent tetanus. I usually get a separate bottle and

fill it up with half Hypericum and half Calendula tincture and call this bottle Hypercal. I use this bottle for making my lotions for wounds on nervy areas. One of the leading symptoms for Hypericum is shooting pains along the nerve path from the injured area.

Treatment

1/. Deal with bleeding and clean wound under running tap or hose water if possible.

2/. Do the final cleaning with Calendula or Hypercal lotion mixed 1 to 20 parts water.

3/. Cover and protect the wound if you think it is necessary.

4/. When wound is dry and healing (if weeping use Hypercal lotion) you can use Calendula cream with maybe Comfrey cream as well for scar prevention or if the wound is healing slowly. You can also medicate a little bit of Calendula cream with Hypericum to make a Hypercal cream for a healing wound giving off nervy pain.

Homoeopathic Treatment

Hypercal - Which is a half and half mixture of Hypericum and Calendula tinctures. you can use this to make lotions when you want the effects of both Calendula and Hypericum. A example on a human would be a infected crushed finger.

Creams - Calendula and Hypericum creams can be used when the healing begins and are applied for the same reasons as the lotions.

Arnica 6 to 30C - For shock, bruised sore pain of the

wound, doesn't like effected area being touched.

Ledum 6 to 30C - Used for puncture wounds, prevents tetanus.

Puncture Wounds

Splinters and accidents from stepping on pins, rusty nails, barbed wire or from tools can be dealt with very effectively with natural remedies.

Herbal Treatment

Hypercal Lotion - Externally use a lotion of Hypercal making sure plenty gets inside the wound so as to prevent tetanus. Other than this treat as a wound.

Homoeopathic Treatment

Arnica 6 to 30C - Can help bring splinters to the surface and deal with any shock.

Hypericum 6 to 30C - Intense pain shoots up from injured parts especially from those in nerve rich areas, if given immediately it can prevent tetanus from developing especially in puncture wounds of the hoofs but it is always best to get a booster shot.

Ledum 6 to 30C - This remedy also prevents tetanus and can be used for the same injuries as Hypericum but with Ledum the part feels cold and is relieved by cold, there is puffiness and a pale mottled appearance.

Herbal Overview Of The Skin

For problems such as Ringworm look to the Anti-Fungal and Anti Biotic herbs, also consider lotions such as Calendula with Garlic and Tea Tree oil in a spray bottle so as to soak a area and for easy application. For the long drawn out chronic diseases of the skin use the Alteratives especially the ones with a strong affinity to the skin such as Sarsaparilla, Burdock, Cleavers and Nettles. The blood cleansers need time to do their work so always consider using them for 3 months as this is the life cycle of the red blood cells so you would of cleaned most of the blood after using them for this time.

Herbal Actions For The Skin

Alterative - Herbs that gradually restore proper function to the body, they increase health and vitality. They were once known as the blood cleansers.

Herbs - Black Cohosh, Blue Flag, Burdock, Cleavers, Chaparral, Echinacea, Fumitory, Garlic, Nettles, Pau D'Arco ,Sarsaparilla, Sweet Violets, Yellow Dock.

Anti-biotic - Echinacea, Garlic, Myrrh, Pau D' Arco, Tea Tree Oil

Anti-fungal - Marigold, Cats Claw, Pau D' Arco, Myrrh, Sweet Violets.

Anti-inflammatory - Helps the body to combat inflammations. Herbs mentioned under demulcents, emollients and vulneraries will often act in this way especially when they are applied externally.

Herbs - Arnica, Blue Flag, Cats Claw, Chaparral ,Chickweed, Cleavers, Cranesbill, Chamomile, Eyebright, Ginger, Golden Rod, Guaiacum, Liquorice, Marshmallow, Marigold, Pau D' Arco, St Johns Wort, Sweet Violets, Witch Hazel.

Astringent - Contracts tissue which in turn reduces discharges, these herbs contain tannins.

Herbs - Agrimony, Bear Berry, Cranesbill, Chaparral, Chickweed, Comfrey, Eyebright, Golden Rod, Hops, Horsetail, Ladys Mantle, Marigold, Marshmallow, Meadowsweet, Myrrh, Nettles, Raspberry, Sage, Rosemary, Slippery Elm, Shepherds Purse, St Johns Wort, Slippery Elm, Thyme, Witch Hazel, Yarrow.

Emollient - Soothing to the skin. Acts externally the way demulcents do internally.

Herbs - Chickweed, Coltsfoot, Comfrey, Fenugreek, Liquorice, Marshmallow, Mullein, Plantain, Slippery Elm.

Parasiticide - Kills parasites and insects.

Herbs - Aniseed, Garlic, Neem, Rosemary,

Vulnerary - Applied externally and aid the body in the healing of wounds and cuts

Herbs - Arnica, Burdock, Chickweed, Comfrey, Cranesbill, Elder, Fenugreek, Garlic, Horsetail, Hyssop, Marigolds, Marshmallow, Mullein, Myrrh, Plantain, Shepherds Purse, Slippery Elm, St Johns Wort, Thyme, Witch Hazel, Yarrow.

The Female Reproductive System

Cystic Ovaries

Associated with the over development of the Graffian Follicle. In animals developing cystic ovary disease, ovulation fails to occur because the egg is not released and the follicle continues to enlarge. Moreover, other follicles may grow and form multiple cysts. The size and form of an affected ovary depends on how extensive the condition is. This condition can lead to one extreme or the other eg never coming to heat or even nymphomania. Between these conditions there could be irregular heat periods. Bitches with this condition may show an uncertain temperament. The problem basically is a massive hormone imbalance which won't go away till the cysts stop developing. The bigger the cyst the more hormones it will be making. There may be a hereditary factor to this disease.

Signs and Symptoms

If the bitch does not cycle there may be one or two cysts present. Symptoms can vary considerably but infertility is the obvious one.

Herbal Treatment

This is difficult to treat so we will start with the basics. Think of starting off with Dong Quai , this is a specific for easing the pain of ovarian cysts but I want to use its blood cleansing properties (Alterative) with those of Burdock which is also Alterative but is also anti-tumor. What I am trying to focus on is cleansing out the womb and blood. We will have to run these herbs for at least 3 months as this is the time it takes for the blood to replace it self-e.g. the blood cycle. Another herb to think of adding to this is Black Cohosh as it is also a Alterative and is also used for pain. Think of using Chaste Tree in about 6 weeks after the first 2 two herbs have had a chance to clean up the area and hopefully reduce the size of the cysts as this will start having a action on the pituitary gland to start sorting out the hormone imbalances. If there is a lot of pain think of Wild Yam.

Homoeopathic Treatment

Apis 6C - One of the main remedies for dropiscal conditions. Used for swelling and puffing up of various parts, edema. Dose 3 time daily for 4 days.

Aurum Mur Nat 6C - When a chronic metritis is suspected and the whitish discharge shows. This remedy has a strong action on growths of the womb and surrounding areas. Ovaries may be indurated. Dose 3 times daily for 4 days.

Colocynth 6C - Nymphomania, multiple small cysts, great abdominal pain especially in the ovary area. Pains are relieved by pressure. Dose night and morning for 1 week.

Platina Met 30C - Nymphomania

Inflammation of the Ovaries

Inflammation of the ovary if present may be suspected by the animal gnawing at the flank or flanks and stretching out the hind legs and there may be a vaginal discharge. Symptoms are very much subjective in this condition.

Herbal Treatment

We really need to know what's causing the inflammation; if it is from a infection then we should give our usual immune boosters Echinacea, Myrrh and Garlic. Black Cohosh and Dong Quai are both female acting herbs that are not only pain killers but are also Alteratives so they will start cleaning up the system as well as relieving the pain. Wild yam is also a good herb for pain in this area. Other herbs to consider are Cramp bark, Angelica, Ladies Mantle, Squaw Vine and Shepherds Purse.

Homoeopathic Treatment

The remedies below all have a action on the ovaries and are worth considering if the ovaries are suspected

Apis Mel 30C - As acute inflammation is usually attended by edema and pain this remedy may be of some help.

Bryonia 6C - The right ovary is more affected with this remedy and the animal will prefer to lie on that side and may be still and quiet. Dose 3 times daily for 2 days.

Cimicifiga 30C - Tenderness over the pelvic area which is worst in the lower left area. There is usually a accompanying muscular weakness and stiffness.

Lachesis 30C - Should be considered if left ovarian trouble is suspected. The skin is often bluish purple in color when this remedy is indicated particularly over the mammary area and in addition throat swellings may be prominent.

Iodum 30C - A suitable remedy for the lean animal with dry coat and exhibiting abnormal appetite. Superficial lymph glands are small and hard and mammary tissue becomes hard and shrunken. the urine assumes a dark yellowish green color.

Lilium Tigrinum 200C - Accompanying signs of uterine inflammation such as discharges etc, discharges only when moving about, has a powerful influence over the pelvic organs, pain in ovaries and down thighs. Dose 3 times daily for 3 days.

Palladium 30C - Right ovary affected with leucorrhoea and flatulence, averse to exercise, pain seems to be relieved after stool and by rubbing. Dose night and morning for one week.

Pulsatilla 30C- The remedy will suit the affectionate bitch which exhibits changeable behavior and sometimes shows a creamy uterine discharge.

Metritis Acute (Inflammation of the Uterus)

Metritis or inflammation of the womb can be acute or chronic. The acute condition is more associated with birth and runs a short course of up to five days. Chief among the causes of this condition is the retained placenta together with infection which gains entrance to the genital tract. In situations other than birth infection can gain entrance to the womb during the heat cycle. This condition is more common in young dogs.

Signs and Symptoms

There is a rise in temperature and the bitch is uneasy and lethargic and may repeatedly lick at her vulva. There may be diarrhea and vomiting along with signs of dehydration. The eyes are sunken and have a anxious expression. Thirst is increased but the appetite is poor or absent. Uterine discharges are present and vary in character from muco-purulent in mild cases to dark brown containing blood stained material in the more severe form.

Herbal Treatment

We will start off by telling you how this problem on the pregnancy side could of probably been avoided in the first place. If the dog was given the herbs Raspberry or Squaw Vine in the last month of pregnancy these herbs would of toned and strengthened the uterus and the problem may of been avoided. At the onset of labor if the herb Golden Seal was used it could of given the dog the extra strength and energy to have a successful and problem free labor, this usually works by making the contractions stronger. When the puppies are born it is usually when they start to suckle that triggers the expulsion of the placenta. Inflammations of the uterus arising from infection should be treated with the main immune boosting herbs mainly Echinacea, Garlic and another good one if you have got it is Myrrh. To these herbs consider adding Ladys Mantle (astringent) Black or Blue Cohosh, or Saw Palmetto. Cleavers could be used as a Alterative for cleaning out the system. A lotion of Calendula could be used to clean the outside area especially if it is red and sore also think of adding Hypericum to the lotion for pain relief.

Homoeopathic Treatment

Treatment should be started as bad signs start to appear after parturition especially after dead pups and a difficult labor.

Aconitum 30C - Should be given at once so as to quickly allay shock, fear and anxiety and regulate the circulation.

Belladonna 30C - Indicated when the animal is hot to touch with a full bounding pulse and dilated pupils. Signs of cerebral excitement may be present with extreme cases convulsions.

Apis Mel 30C - Also useful in the early stages when a degree of edema will be present in the uterine lining.

Lillum Tig 30C - A good general remedy for uterine congestion leading to blood stained discharges and straining in the pelvic region.

Secale 6C - Hemorrhages are present when this remedy is considered, the blood is fluid and dark, the patient is cadaverous looking with cold extremities which are deficient in blood supply.

Sabina 6C- Useful when the condition is associated with the retention of the afterbirth or miscarriage especially in those cases showing blood stained discharges. Give every hour for 6 doses.

Pyrogen 1M - This nosode is indicated when a weak thready pulse alternates with a high temperature or vice versa. The most useful remedy in septic conditions. Give every 2 hours for 4 doses.

The Vagina and Vulva

The most common condition here is inflammation of the vulva and vagina both frequently being together at the same time. It is important to find the cause and if it is infection it must be dealt with fast so as to stop it from going deeper in the body.

Signs and Symptoms

Redness and swelling accompanied by edema. Examination of the mucous membrane inside reveals the lining reddened and painful. A clear discharge may be present and in neglected cases may become purulent. The bitch will be seen licking the vulva and at the end of urination there may be straining. If not treated a infection could travel deeper and follow the ureters and infect the kidneys.

Herbal Treatment

Read the herbal section on cystitis and especially take note of the urinary antiseptics. If infection is present or even suspected give our usual immune boosters Echinacea, Myrrh and Garlic. Other good herbs to consider for this area are Angelica, Black and Blue cohosh, Cramp bark, Dong Quai and Squaw Vine. Astringents are used to reduce the flow of discharges and to tone tissue, common astringents for this area are Shepherds Purse, Ladys Mantle and Raspberry. Remember it may not be wise to stop discharge as this is the body's way of getting rid of rubbish.

Homoeopathic Treatment

Antimonium Crud 6C - The parts are excessively itchy and a uterine discharge of a creamy nature is usually present. Skin eruptions of a pimply nature may accompany the condition.

Apis Mel 30C - Will help control the edematous swelling and remove the stinging pains which are usually present. This remedy should be given as early as possible when swelling is first noticed.

Rhus Tox 6C - The vaginal mucous membrane is intensely red and itching and the swelling is severe. Blistery skin eruptions may be present together with stiffness of movement which decreases with exercise.

Cantharis 6C - Indicated when there is severe straining during and after the passage of urine. The bitch may exhibit frenzied sexual behavior. Itching of genital area is intense.

Helonias 30C - Fever, itching and swelling are associated with this remedy, together with sacral weakness which produces a dragging movement on attempting to rise. Catarrhal exudation is usually present.

Nit Acid 30C - A remedy where inflammation affects the mucous membranes near the body's orifices with or without ulceration. Discharge may have blood in it. There is sometimes diarrhea of a slimy nature accompanying the condition.

Pregnancy

Herbal Treatment

Raspberry leaf is the most important herbal aid to a easy birth as it tones the uterine muscles, is very high in vitamins and minerals and increases and enriches the milk production. Another important reason for using Raspberry is because of its high astringency which gives us protection against excessive bleeding. Raspberry should be given to all breeders especially the ones that have had difficult births before and those that have had retained after birth before. Give Raspberry before pregnancy and in the last month before birth. At the onset of labor if the herb Golden Seal was used it could of given the dog the extra strength and energy to have a successful and problem free labor, this usually works by making the contractions stronger. When the puppies are born it is usually when they start to suckle that triggers the expulsion of the placenta. Herbs to think of to increase the milk production are Fenugreek, and Fennel.

Homoeopathic Treatment

Viburnum Opulis - A remedy for use in the early stages of pregnancy up to one month to 6 weeks. Helps to eliminate the tendency to early miscarriage. Give 30C three times per week for 4 weeks.

Caulophyllum - This remedy is used for the latter stages. Helps to ensure a trouble free birth and tones up the uterus for easy expulsion of the afterbirth. Give 30C three times per week for the last 4 weeks. If the last stage of labor is delayed or weak this remedy should be given again to help speed up normal contractions.

Arnica 30C - This can be used at the time of birthing and given for a few days after as it will help with the bruising and swelling and is good for shock. Give 3 times a day.

BellisPerennis 30C - If the birthing was prolonged or severe give this remedy along with Arnica.

Helps to eliminate the tendency to early miscarriage. Give 30C three times per week for 4 weeks. \

Haemorrhage
Herbal Treatment
Astringents are the main herbs that you use to stop bleeding. Two of the strongest ones are Shepherds Purse and Cranesbill. Make a 1 to 10 lotion of either of these herbs and if bleeding cannot be controlled use a small syringe without the needle to gently inject into the womb, hopefully this will spasm the ends of the bleeding vessels and stop the flow of blood. Give a strong dose internally as well.

Homoeopathic Treatment
Ipecacuanah 6C - Blood accumulates in the uterus and is then expelled in a bright red flood. Give every hour for 5 doses.

Crotalus 1M - If the blood comes away as a steady drip. Give every hour for 4 doses.

Hammamelis 30C - Dark blood indicating a venous origin will need this remedy. Give 1 dose every 2 hours up to 5 times.

Secale 30C - Very stringy blood indicates this remedy. Give 1 dose every 2 hours up to 5 times.

Acute Mastitis

Inflammation of the Mammary Gland. The cause can be a combination of factors such as exposure to cold winds and wet weather, injuries from blows and sharp objects, and bacterial infections caught from others or as a result of poor hygiene. Mastitis can occur anytime during lactation but is frequently seen after birth.

Signs and Symptoms

This condition is sometimes seen after parturition when one or more glands become swollen, hot and tender to touch, the milk becomes curdled and yellow after a while and in neglected cases discoloration of the mammary region occurs. The bitch is obviously in pain and discomfort and has an anxious expression. There may be a increase in temperature and the dog will go off food. Sometimes the dog tries to keep the legs from contacting the udder and as a result may walk with a different gait and stand with the rear legs apart. This is a serious condition that needs immediate treatment also the puppies must be stopped from using that teat as the infected milk will cause them problems sometimes death may result.

Herbal Treatment

Humans sometimes use a cabbage leaf poultice for this condition, get some cabbage leafs and pound them so they are bruised all over and apply to the affected area, I'll leave you to figure out how to do this as I aren't all that sure myself as usually women use a oversized bra to hold the leaves in place. Photolacca tincture in small doses is the main herb for mastitis though I believe the Homoeopathic potency is far better and faster acting then the tincture. To the Homoeopathic Dose you could make a lotion of Photolacca but make it a very mild lotion as this is a strong remedy so make it about 1 to 20 in strength. The main immune boosting herbs should also be used these are Echinacea, Garlic and Myrrh as well as the Alteratives such as Cleavers. . Wood Sage (has a affinity to the udder) was also given with this treatment but is now very difficult to find. Wood Sage can be made into a lotion and applied to the udder.

Homoeopathic Treatment

Aconitum 12C - Should be given in the early stages if possible. It will reduce anxiety and help calm the patient.

Arnica 30C - Indicated when mastitis develops as a result of injury to the mammary tissue, blood may be present in the milk. Dose 3 times daily for 3 days.

Belladonna 200C - Indicated when the glands are swollen, hot and tense, dilated pupils and a full and bounding pulse are present, increased sensitivity or excessive excitability may be seen.

Apis Mel 30C - Where edema and stinging pain is present.

Phytolacca 30C - This is a valuable remedy as it has a selective action on the mammary gland. The inflammation may take the form of nodular patches of hard tissue while clots in the milk usually disappear under its influence.

Bryonia 30C - Useful remedy when the gland is excessively hard, there may be attendant constipation and respiratory upset such as pleurisy, general stiffness of limbs is present.

Hepar Sulph 200C - The bitch exhibits aversion to touch indicating excessive tenderness and pain. Mammary secretion is probably thin and purulent.

Ipecac 30C - This is a useful remedy for controlling intra-mammary bleeding which results in pink milk. Dose 3 times daily for 3 days.

Teats Sore Or Damaged

The delicate tissues of the teat sometimes become chapped and develop deep fissures.

Symptoms - Damage or redness is seen and or the dog winces and will not tolerate the feeding.

Herbal Treatment - Juliette de Bairacli Levy recommends to treat alternately with warm almond oil as a salve and bathed with a brew of equal parts elder blossom and marshmallow. Raw cucumber juice has been effective. I would use Calendula and Hypericum Lotion (1 to 10) as this is a great healer of all wounds and also helps to relieve the pain.

Herbal Overview Of The Reproductive System

Herbs to think of when a miscarriage is suspected are False Unicorn Root, Ladys Slipper, Blue Cohosh, Black Haw, Wild Yam, and Cramp Bark. The main herbs to think of for pregnancy are Raspberry, Squaw Vine and Shepherds Purse. Below are some of the actions to consider for this system. In the Astringents the herbs underlined are the best to use to stop bleeding. Use the Alteratives for Chronic diseases of this system and maybe add some of the Emmenagogues to them after reading up on the individual herbs and adding the one that works in the direction you want.

Herbal Actions For The Reproductive System

Alterative - Herbs that gradually restore proper function to the body, they increase health and vitality. They were once known as the blood cleansers.

Herbs - Black Cohosh, Dong Quai, Damiana, Skullcap.

Anti-biotic - Chaparral, Echinacea, Garlic, Myrrh, Pau D' Arco, Reshi.

Anti-fungal - Marigold, Cats Claw, Pau D' Arco, Myrrh, Sweet Violets.

Anti-inflammatory - Helps the body to combat inflammations. Herbs mentioned under demulcents, emollients and vulneraries will often act in this way especially when they are applied externally.

Herbs - Cranesbill, Chamomile, Eyebright, Feverfew, Ginger, Golden Rod, Ladys Mantle, Licorice, Marshmallow, Meadowsweet, Marigold, Pau D' Arco, St Johns Wort, Witch Hazel.

Anti-Tumor - Burdock, Cleavers, Reshi, Shitake, Sweet Violets.

Antispasmodic - Prevents or eases spasms and cramps.

Herbs - Aniseed, Angelica, Black Cohosh, Chamomile, Fennel, Hyssop, Motherwort, Rosemary, Rue, Sage, Skullcap, St Johns Wort, Thyme, Valerian, Vervain.

Anti-viral - Astragalus, Cats claw, Echinacea, Garlic, Myrrh?, Shitake, St Johns Wort, Pau D'Arco.

Astringent - Contracts tissue which in turn reduces discharges, these herbs contain tannins.

Herbs - Agrimony, Cranesbill, Eyebright, Golden Rod, Ladys Mantle, Marigold, Raspberry, Shepherds Purse, St Johns Wort, Witch Hazel.

Emmenagogue - Stimulates and normalizes the menstrual flow, tonics for the female reproductive system.

Herbs - Black Cohosh, Chamomile, Fenugreek, Gentian, Ginger, Juniper, Ladys Mantle, Marigold, Motherwort, Parsley, Penny Royal, Peppermint, Parsley, Raspberry, Sage, Rosemary, Rue, Shepherds Purse, St Johns Wort, Tansy, Thyme, Valerian, Vervain, Wormwood, Yarrow.

Galactagogue - Helps increase the flow of milk in females.

Herbs - Aniseed, Fennel, Fenugreek, Milk Thistle, Raspberry, Vervain.

Notes

Serious Infectious Diseases

Distemper

This disease is of widespread occurrence and though the primary cause is a virus it is often complicated with secondary opportunistic bacterial problems. The virus is airborne and other animals such as foxes, weasels and ferrets can carry and transmit the disease. Young animals in the puppy stage are more at risk than the older dog.

Signs and Symptoms

In the very young pup the only signs of the disease may be diarrhea which may be blood stained and there is no appetite. Older puppies and dogs over four months of age get a fever and a temperature 3 to 4 degrees above normal. In the classical form the nose is dry and hot and the eyes have a anxious look. The fever is followed by a discharge from the eyes and nose which is at first watery and clear but latter becomes cloudy containing mucous and sometimes purulent material. Respiratory involvement starts with a soft moist cough. Other signs can be a harsh dry skin showing a papular or vesicular rash on the abdomen and inner flanks, diarrhea usually foul smelling and blood stained is usually present also.

If the disease is allowed to run its course or early treatment has been ineffective pneumonia develops and may take a severe form with rust colored sputum and nasal discharge. If the animal survives this we move on to nervous system involvement ranges from muscular twitching and chorea affecting cranial or peripheral nerves in milder cases to convulsions which may become progressively worse the longer the animal lives. The spinal cord may become more deeply affected resulting in paralysis of varying degrees. Involvement of the nervous system is usually accompanied by a thickening or induration of the foot pads.

Herbal Treatment.

With infectious diseases as fast acting and as serious as this use high doses of Vitamin C immediately, if you have it in liquid form such as Troys a 8cc dose intramuscularly should be given for the average size dog if not you can give it in Sodium Ascorbate Powder form at about 10 grams a day for the medium sized dog, you can mix the powder with water and gently syringe the liquid into the dogs mouth 3 times a day. It would be best to fast the dog especially at the beginning stages and it is not wise to give a dog food while they have a fever so try to wait till the fever breaks, meanwhile you could give the dog honey and water so they remain hydrated and have some nutrition. Use the immune boosting herbs Echinacea, Garlic and Myrrh constantly throughout the illness and add to them other herbs as the symptoms change. See the different chapters and try to match herbs to the new symptoms you are seeing. Yarrow would be the first herb to add to the immune boosters as this is one of the main herbs that we use in fevers and would also help to fight the infection and act on the dysentery. Try when you select your herbs to get them to overlap and cover other symptoms in there actions as I have done with Yarrow.

Homoeopathic Treatment

Homeopathy has much to offer in the treatment of distemper and we can easily match our remedies to suit each stage of the disease. In the following treatment is laid out in the different stages.

The First Stages

Aconitum 30C - Give this remedy at the first signs of the disease, the expression will be anxious and there may be shivering or other signs of shock present. This remedy given promptly could abort the disease. It should be given at half hourly intervals for a total of 6 doses.

Ferrum Phos 6X - Useful in the early stages especially if the animal is of a sensitive or nervous disposition, anxiety is not present, the throat is red and inflamed and there may be a accompanying nose bleed.

Belladonna 30C - The animal shows dilated pupils and may be excitable, there is full bounding pulse and the skin is hot and dry.

Stage of Coryza with Lachrymation

Arsen Alb 1M - Restlessness is the keynote for this remedy, the animal sips water frequently but only takes small amounts, symptoms are worse towards midnight, discharges from the eyes and nose are acrid and excoriate the skin.

Merc Corr 30C - Severe lachrymation which may become purulent showing as yellow blobs in the corners of the eyes, symptoms usually worse from sunset to sunrise.

Pulsatilla 30C - Discharges are catarrhal or bland and frequently profuse, is especially suited to the animal which has a timid or gentle disposition.

Stage of Respiratory Involvement Consider the following. Refer to Respiratory in Borickes Materia Medica. - Antimonium Tart ,Ipecacuanha 30C ,Bryonia 30C, Lycopodium 30C ,Phosphorus

Stage of Gastro-Intestinal Involvement Refer to Stomach and Abdomen in Borickes Marteria Medica Arsen Alb, Merc Corr 30C, Baptisia 30C, China Officinalis 30C.

Stage of Skin Involvement refer to skin in Borickes Materia Medica - Antimonium Crud 6C,Arsen Alb 30C
Stage of Nervous System Involvement, Gelsemium 30C, Belladonna 1M, Conium 30C, Causticum 6C

Stage of eye Involvement usually inflammations or ulcerations see eye in Borickes Materia Medica -
Aurum Met 30C, Merc Corr 30C,Euphrasia 6C, Argent Nit 6C, Pulsatilla 30C - Externally all cases should be bathed with a 1/10 solution of Calendula and Hypericum repeated a few times each day.

Parvovirus Disease

This is a viral infection that mainly affects puppies though older animal can be effected. The virus is strong and can live outside the body for up to a year. Infection occurs when the dogs takes the virus in the mouth. Rapid death can follow infection in the young chiefly from dehydration and involvement of the heart muscle. Diagnosis is made from a sample of faeces.

Signs and Symptoms

The disease has a sudden onset with the patient first showing signs of depression and anorexia, then vomiting and diarrhea, the faeces being watery and foul smelling and having a orange yellow color. Blood may be present in both the vomit and faeces. The vomiting may be difficult to stop and dehydration is especially marked in puppies. Dehydration is an important factor in this disease and many dogs have died in 2 to 3 days just from this.

The temperature may only be slightly raised and the mouth may show small vesicles which on rupturing leaving a raw bleeding surface.

Herbal Treatment

With infectious diseases as fast acting and as serious as this use high doses of Vitamin C immediately, if you have it in liquid form such as Troys a 8cc dose intramuscularly should be given for the average size dog if not you can give it in Sodium Ascorbate Powder form at about 10 grams a day for the medium sized dog, you can mix the powder with water and gently syringe the liquid into the dogs mouth 3 times a day. It would be best to fast the dog especially at the beginning, meanwhile you could give the dog honey (raw for its antibiotic effect) and water so they remain hydrated and have some nutrition. Dehydration is the biggest killer in this disease so go to the chemist and get some rehydration powder and add this to the honey, Vit C water etc. Use the immune boosting herbs Echinacea, Garlic and Myrrh constantly throughout the illness and add to them other herbs as the symptoms change. If the dog is vomiting the herbal tinctures can be added to the water and honey used for rehydration and maybe add Meadowsweet and or Peppermint so as to try and control the vomiting. Bear in mind that it may not be wise to stop the vomiting and diarrhea to soon as it would be best to let nature get the toxins out of the system as fast as possible but of course you cannot let the condition go on forever. Refer to the Digestive System to match symptoms and find other herbs.

Homoeopathic Treatment

Try to get the disease Nosode.

Aconitum 30C - Should be given as soon as possible, one dose every hour for four doses, use this remedy for the sudden onset of any acute disease.

Arsen Alb 30C - This remedy is the main one to control diarrhea in the acute stages and again frequent doses are necessary.

Antimonium Tart 30C - The tongue is coated with red edges, swallowing is difficult and is accompanied by retching and vomiting, rumbling of intestines may be heard preceding stool which is accompanied by straining, the stools themselves being watery with shreds of mucous.

Crotalus Horr 30C - If there is considerable blood being lost in the faeces it may be necessary to use this remedy in addition to those already mentioned as it is one of the main ant hemorrhagic remedies we have and frequent doses are advisable.

Iris Versicolor 30C - This is a useful remedy to follow after acute symptoms have been controlled by the previous remedies.

Ipecacuanha 30C - Retching and vomiting may lead to collapse. The vomit is slimy and may be continuous. Slimy diarrhea possibly blood stained may be present also. There may also be reflex respiratory symptoms such as coughing and difficulty in breathing.

Leptospirosis - Weil's Disease

This is a bacterial disease which is spread by contaminated urine and can also be caught by a contamination of a wound. In dogs it was once known a Lamp Posts disease for obvious reasons. The organisms invade the bloodstream for a week or more and then attack the kidneys. The disease may take various forms ranging from acute to chronic. This disease may cross to humans.

Signs and Symptoms

The onset of symptoms in the acute form can be quite

sudden and the animal is seen vomiting and passing loose motions. Loss of appetite and a dehydrated appearance set in. There could be a temperature of 103 to 105 on the first day dropping the next. Gastrointestinal involvement takes the form of bile stained vomiting together with dark brown or blood stained stools, the presence of bile in the stools may give it a green tinge, pain is evident on abdominal palpation , the coat becomes harsh and dry and walking becomes difficult with signs of stiffness being apparent over the sacral area. Ulceration of the mucous membranes in the mouth is a common feature and there may be signs of jaundice. With the respiratory system there may be signs of coryza with frequent coughing, the urine becomes dark and bile stained.

Herbal Treatment

This disease can cross over to people so isolate the animal and take protective hygiene measures and keep the kids away. With infectious diseases as fast acting and as serious as this use high doses of Vitamin C immediately, if you have it in liquid form such as Troys a 8cc dose intramuscularly should be given for the average size dog if not you can give it in Sodium Ascorbate Powder form at about 10 grams a day for the medium sized dog, you can mix the powder with water and gently syringe the liquid into the dogs mouth 3 times a day. It would be best to fast the dog especially at the beginning stages and it is not wise to give a dog food while they have a fever so try to wait till the fever breaks, meanwhile you could give the dog honey and water so they remain hydrated and have some nutrition. Use the immune boosting herbs Echinacea, Garlic and Myrrh constantly throughout the illness and add to them other herbs as the symptoms change. This disease seems to cause ulceration and bleeding throughout the digestive tract and liver problems so we shall concentrate our treatment on these areas, when you give your water and honey we can add to this Slippery elm powder but not too much as we want to keep the liquid still very liquid, this will act as a mild astringent (helps to stop bleeding) and a demulcent (soothing) as well as supplying nutrition other herbs to look at here are Cranesbill, Comfrey Licorice and Meadowsweet. For the liver look at the Herbs Dandelion and Milk Thistle.

Homoeopathic Treatment

Aconitum 12X - Give this remedy at the first signs of the disease, the expression will be anxious and there may be shivering or other signs of shock present. This remedy given promptly could abort the disease.

Arsen Alb 30C - Could help control the gastro intestinal problems and could be of value in helping overcome dehydration.

Merc Corr 30C - Important remedy once ulceration of the buccal mucous membranes develop, also indicated to control mucous and blood stained diarrhea.

Baptisia 30C - A remedy which may be needed to

combat prostration and muscular soreness. Putrid excretions and bad breath indicate its use. In the classical case this remedy may be better than any other.

Phosphorus 30C - Will help the coughing associated with the respiratory involvement and should have a beneficial effect on the liver leading to a reduction in the vomiting.

Lycopodium 1M - The chronic case showing wasting and no appetite will be helped by this remedy as it has a long term beneficial action on the liver.

Herbal Supplement
Introduction To Herbal Medicine

Herbal Medicine has been in use and developed continuously since the beginning of time. It mainly evolved from observations from what plants did and the affects they had on people along with their animals. There is also what they call the Doctrine of Signatures which works like this, that flower really looks like an eye, maybe it helps sore eyes. I'll give it a try as my eyes are so sore and red. You know my eye really feels a lot better now, I think I will call that plant Eye Bright (Euphrasia) and tell my friends all about it especially my Dad who gets sore eyes to. In this way hundreds of plants were identified that have a medical action and no doubt there were also a lot of casualties.

The next great leap in herbal medicine was the Roman Empire of 2000 years ago. The Great Armies of Rome all had their own Medical Corps with Doctors, Battle Surgeons and Orderlies. It was these men who already had the knowledge of the Greeks that started to put together the best medical manuals in the world while at the same time started developing and using medical instruments and tools some of which are still used today. As the Romans conquered the known world more medicines and knowledge were found and assimilated.

The next great leap was modern Chemistry which allowed us to see exactly what herbs were made up of and what parts of the herb causes its medical action.

Drug companies have made billions of Dollars from this information as they find the main active ingredient and then make a synthetic version of it, one good example that we all know of is Valium which is the synthetic version of the active ingredient from the herb Valerian. Leaving aside the Drug Companies let's see how Chemistry changed the way that modern herbalists think. Modern science allows us to now know what Actions our herbs perform on the body so we shall carry on using Valerian as a example and see what Medical Actions Valerian has on the body.

The Actions of Valerian are Sedative, Hypnotic (sleep inducing), Anti Spasmodic (stops twitches, cramps etc.), Hypotensive (lowers Blood Pressure) and Carminative (calms and relaxes the tummy). Herbalists call Valerian the Herbal Tranquillizer and if you look at the above you can see why for if you can't sleep and your blood pressures up along with a gurgling tummy and an eye constantly twitching you definitely need to be calmed down.

The modern herbalist is trained to think in actions. There are many reasons for this but the main ones are to stop them from just using a handful of their favorite herbs and to train the mind to work in the method of thinking in actions that are needed. If we start thinking in the actions that are needed for a patient it makes us consider the problem in far more depth than just using our favorite herb and it forces our thinking to be far more holistic by taking in consideration the whole of the patient not just the part or the system we wish to treat.

Let's take a look at thinking in actions. The animal has a cough, but when it coughs it can't stop and the cough sounds a bit like whooping cough. The animal also sounds a little hoarse and the temperature is also elevated. The actions that come into mind for this are expectorant for the cough, anti-spasmodics for the whooping quality of the cough and demulcents to sooth the sore throat. These are the obvious actions and we can add many more if we wish such as immune boosters for acute diseases, diaphoretics to reduce the temperature and prevent a fever and the list goes on. Next we look at how Herbal Actions are used in making Herbal Formulas.

Another point to make before we go to the formula making is that Professional Herbalists use Herbs in the form of Tinctures (water and alcohol solutions) as this allows them to mix formulas in any proportions that they like and also allows long term storage without spoiling.

Making Herbal Formulas

You should never have more the 5 Herbs in a herbal formula otherwise you start to loose track of what you are doing and how the formula is changing the symptoms. Always try to keep things simple. One of the herbs in the formula is used to force the formula into the body, to keep it simple we will only use three; they are Licorice, Ginger and Cayenne.

As an example let's use a animal with a cough. After

further study of the case we decide that this is a Acute Disease for it came on quick and is fast acting not slow like a Chronic Disease. Listening to the animals cough we decide that it is a dry cough and upon looking at the animal's nose we can't see any mucus. Let's list the actions to consider.

Expectorants - Licorice, Aniseed, Fennel, Garlic and Mullein

Antispasmodics - Aniseed and Fennel

Demulcents - Licorice and Coltsfoot

Immune Boosters - Echinacea

Anti-Bacterial and Virals - Garlic and Echinacea

Out of the above I would choose Licorice, Echinacea, Garlic, Aniseed and Fennel. I would make the formula in this strength.

Formula
Licorice - 20%
Garlic - 15%
Echinacea - 15%
Aniseed - 30%
Fennel - 20%

Look these herbs up in the herbal and consider why I used them, there are three obvious ones for Licorice alone with the first being to force the assimilation of the formula into the body, second is its expectorant action and third is its demulcent action in case the throat is sore and raw. Next time you see a little kid eating heaps of licorice get them to open their mouth and look at their tongue which will be going black from the Licorice along with the throat etc. and know that you are looking at the demulcent action of Licorice working by coating and soothing.

The most important reason that you use the Actions Method for Herbal Prescribing is so that you can concentrate the Actions which are most needed for example, if it's a Bacterial infection concentrate on the Anti Bacterials, if it's a Viral infection concentrate on the Anti Virals, hopefully you are now beginning to see the importance of working in actions for if you don't concentrate a large part of the battle on the causes you may have lost the battle from the start.

Read through all the Actions listed in Herbal Actions at the end of each body system in the book and then do a study in depth of at least five Actions of your choice making the first two the Anti-Bacterials and Anti-Virals. Start trying to train your mind into thinking in Actions.

How To Make Herbal Tinctures

Tinctures are made by steeping the Herb plant material in a mixture of alcohol and water. Alcohol is usually always used at strength of 45%. The alcohol in this mixture will extract all the essential oils from the herb while the water will extract all that is water soluble, so between the both we are getting most of the medicinal properties out of the herb.

The proportions of herb to liquid are usually 1 part

herb to 5 parts liquid. So find a suitable container (I use a big one liter preserving jar with a good sealing lid) and put into it 100grams of your chosen herb and to that add 500mls of our 45% solution of alcohol. Seal the lid and shake well for about a minute. Leave the jar on the window sill so the sun can shine on the jar for two weeks. The jar must be shaken for at least a minute every day.

After 2 weeks open and filter the contents of the jar. I use a large pouring jug into which I place a funnel and then place a coffee filter in the funnel and pour the jar contents through the funnel being careful not to let to much herb spill into the filter and block it up. When you get to the bottom of the jar you can crush the herb in your fist so as to extract the last of the liquid.

After this is completed you then get your chosen storage bottle, put a funnel into its neck followed by a coffee filter and then filter the jug into the bottle. Remember the solution should always be double filtered

Next we label the bottle, put the date, name and proportions e.g. 1 to 5 also state the recommended dose. Store in a cool and dark place. Most Professional Homoeopaths and Herbalists have access to pure alcohol so for them it is fairly easy to make tinctures while for the lay person they will probably have a hard time. A alternative is to use Vodka as strong as you can find it or find away to twist the authorities arm into giving alcohol at 45%. Don't even try to get pure alcohol as it is dangerous and can turn people blind and they won't give it to you.

How To Make Infusions

Infusions are a bit like making a cup of tea except we don't use milk. Infusions are used for the soft parts of the herb such as the flowers, leaves and fine twigs. The proportions for infusions are 1 to 20 eg 1 part herb to 20 parts water. Infusions are used for the more water soluble herbs. Infusions can be made from a single herb or from a combination of herbs and may be drunk hot or cold. The water should be just off the boil before being poured on the herb and if you are making an infusion of a herb strong in essential oils such as Peppermint always cover the top of the cup to stop the essential oils from escaping in steam while the infusion is brewing. Allow up to 10 minutes to brew. It is best to make herbal teas fresh each day. You can experiment on yourself by getting Chamomile and Peppermint tea bags from the supermarket. Use honey as a sweetener.

How To Make Decoctions

Decoctions are used for the more hard woody substances of the herb such as barks, berries or roots. The process of decoction is far more vigorous then infusion as it involves heating the plant material in cold water, bringing it to the boil and simmering for 20 to 40 minutes. The finished ratio for decoctions is again 1 part herb to 20 parts water; remember to add more water at the beginning so you wind up with the

1 to 20 after steam loss. This form of preparation is no good for the herbs that are high in essential oils as these will all be lost in the steam.

How To Make Poultices

Poultices are used to sooth, irritate or draw impurities from the skin so choose your required plants by the actions you need. A Poultice is used to apply a remedy to the skin with moist heat and slight pressure. To prepare a poultice bruise or crush the fresh medicinal parts of the herb you are using into a pulpy mass and add a little hot water if needed. If using dried herb moisten the material by mixing with a hot soft adhesive substance such as moist flower and cornmeal or as they did in the past a mixture of bread and milk. This can be done to the fresh herb if you want as well. For ease of application to the skin it is best to spread the mixture on cheese cloth and fold to the appropriate size or shape required. The cloth also helps by retaining the moisture and even allows you to tie it gently the affected area. Moisten the cloth with hot water periodically when and if needed. Hot water bottles can also be used to keep the poultice warm. Always keep some cloth between the skin when using irritant plants such as mustard and always wash the skin thoroughly after use.

Dosage For Forms Of Herbal Medicines

Herbs can be given to animals in several different

forms depending on what best suites the herb, the ailment, and the condition of the animal and of what is available at the time and then most importantly the expense. I prefer using liquid to medicate in tinctures, extracts or infusion form even though there can be some controversy over the alcohol. The reason for this is that liquid spreads through the intestines a greater distance then the dry form which insures maximum absorption and uptake. Juliette de Bairacli Levy uses mainly infusions made from one handful of the fresh herb or 2 heaped tablespoons of the dried herb to one pint of cold water slowly heated and simmered for a while not boiled. Her dose is based on a Cocker Spaniel sized dog and is two level tablespoons of infusion morning and night. Smaller dogs get less and bigger dogs more. She uses infusions because cellulose is not easily digested in carnivore animals though she does use some herbal powders. For the same size dog that she used as a example I would consider using Tincture form at about 5 drops diluted with water three times a day but always go by what the maker of the tincture says because all herbs are not the same strength some are very strong with a good example being Poke Root.

Herbal Extract - Are alcohol based and about the strongest herbal preparation you can get as they nearly extract everything from the herb. Generally the strength is every ml should be equivalent to one gram of the herb. Used and dosed the same as tinctures but the dose will always be less than what is used in a tincture. From this try to work out if the extra price is worth it. Supplier should give dosage.

Tincture - Is a weaker then Herbal Extracts but also made from alcohol. Dilute the appropriate number of drops in water for treatment. Supplier should give dosage.

Infusion - A infusion is like making a cup of tea out of the flowers and leaves and other soft parts of the herb. Add boiling water and cover so as all the essential oils don't escape in the steam and leave for 20 minutes.

Decoction - Usually made from the root, bark or seed and is simmered for a while to extract the medicinal properties. Usually dosed the same as infusions.

Powdered - These are usually made from roots and bark and given in doses from a teaspoon to tablespoon. These can also be infused and turned into a tea.

Note - Always be guided by the recommended dose of the individual herb instead of working in generals.

Calculating Correct Herbal Doses For Animals

Below is a general rule for doses in animals, always use commonsense and less is better than to much.

Cats - 1/8 to 1/6 the dose for an adult human.

Dogs - Correspond to adult human dose according to weight.

Horse - 8 to 16 times the dose for an adult human.

Goats - 2 times the dose for an adult human.

Sheep - 1 1/2 times the dose for an adult human.

Cow - 12 to 24 times the dose for an adult human.

Swine - 1 to 3 times the dose for an adult human.

Not all herbs are of the same strength so for this reason it is a good idea to always look at the human dose and if this dose seems to be lower than normal, do your research into why. It might be a good idea to have a look at the herb Poke Root just to see what a strong herb looks like and can do.

Notes

Good Cat And Dog Herbs

These are herbs that are fairly safe for use and have a long history of dog use and most importantly they should be easy for you to find. There are lots more herbs that you can use but get used to these ones first and slowly expand.

Agrimony

Actions - Astringent, cholagogue, diuretic, vulnerary, tonic

Used as a remedy for jaundice, it should be given to fasting animal as a drench or finely cut and mixed with bran, it is also a valuable astringent to stem bleeding and is a remedy for sore throats. Sprains are aided by a lotion made by boiling one handful of chopped Agrimony in one quart of brew made from wheaten bran. The combination of astringency and of bitter tonic properties make this a powerful herb for the digestive system. This is a good and gentle remedy for the young.

Uses - Diarrhea in the young, mucous colitis, spring tonic, indigestion, urinary incontinence and cystitis, as a gargle for sore throats and laryngitis and as a ointment or lotion for wounds and bruises.

For Cats and Dogs - Sore throats, Tonsillitis, infections of the mouth, Ailments of the lungs, stomach, liver kidney and bladder particularly cirrhosis of the liver and jaundice, it helps rheumatism, poor digestion and back pain and is excellent for enlargement of the heart and disorders

of the spleen. Infusions, decoctions, ointments.
Cautions - Not to be used during Pregnancy

Alfalfa

Known also as Lucerne. Rich in nitrates and vitamins is a good tonic food and a kidney cleanser. Excellent for all animals and poultry. It is a healthy and nutritious source of chlorophyll, beta carotene, calcium, and the vitamins D, E and K. Fodder, tonic, nervine, aids in healing allergies, arthritis, morning sickness, peptic ulcers, stomach ailments and bad breath, removes poisons from the body, neutralizes acids, is a excellent blood purifier and thinner, improves appetite and aids in the assimilation of protein, calcium and other nutrients.

Dogs - 2 teaspoons of fresh chopped alfalfa sprouts with daily meal as a natural enzyme for good digestion.

Calendula

Actions - Anti-inflammatory, astringent, vulnerary, anti-fungal, cholagogue, emmenagogue.
A good cancer herb which also brings great relief to inflammation of the liver. It purifies the blood so stimulating the circulation and bringing swift healing to wounds. One of the best Vulnerary herbs for external use.

Uses - Cuts, grazes, infected sores, fungal infections, any skin inflammations, regulates the oil production of the skin so is good for acne, to stop bleeding, bruises and sprains, skin ulcers and minor burns and scolds, healing, soothing, anti-microbial. Use as a lotion to clean wounds, one of our main germacides for wounds and if Hypericum is added to the lotion you may prevent tetanus as well.

Caution - Calendula closes wounds rapidly so make sure they are very clean and no foreign bodies remain.

Chamomile

Actions - Stomachic, antispasmodic, anti-allergy, sedative, anti-inflammatory, carminative, analgesic and anti-septic.

It is a famed blood cleanser and pain reducer, reduces tumors (poultice), remedy for female ailments, inflamed gums, use for blood and skin disorders, aches and pains, external and internal inflammations, delayed menstruation, acid uterus and all female ailments, cleanser and toner of the digestive tract, expels worms and parasites, improves and helps appetite. This herb is also anti-allergy.

Uses - Indigestion, colic, diarrhea, teething children, anxiety, insomnia, **nervous upsets,** slowing down hyperactive children, flatulence. Good all round tonic for the nervous system especially for nervous animals.

Cats and Dogs - Good for kittens and puppies, administer in all cases of stomach pain, wind, upsets, gastritis, restlessness and fever. Can be given also for all abdominal and uterine disorders, inflammation of the testicles, wounds, toothaches, eruptions and as a steam bath for colds and feline respiratory diseases. Fevers, back and rheumatic pains are eased by the tea and regular massages with the oil. The infusion is good for nervous disorders and a tonic for kidney and urinary tract problems

Cat Nip - Cat Mint - Carminative, antispasmodic, diaphoretic, sedative, astringent.

Cats eat the plant and give themselves a massage in it in order to benefit from its medicinal properties. It will sometimes cause cats to grow pensive and dreamy. It is a digestive plant that will heal colic, flatulence and internal inflammation. It stops coughs and is a gentle efficient pain killer.

Cleavers

Actions - Alterative, diuretic, anti-inflammatory, tonic, astringent, lymphatic tonic.

A lymphatic tonic with alterative and diuretic actions which can be used in a wide range of problems where the lymphatic system is involved. The plant is very rich in minerals and silica, gives good strong texture to the hair of animals and the shells of eggs. All animals eat it and poultry especially seek it hence its popular name of goose grass. Good for skin ailments.

Uses - Tonic, eczema, abscesses and tumors, cancerous growths, swollen glands, tonsillitis, psoriasis, cystitis.

Cats and Dogs - Cleavers is a great purifier of the kidneys, pancreas and spleen. Disorders of the uterus, the lymphatic system and the skin are helped by this herb. The fresh juice applied to cases of feline acne and eczema quickly alleviates the problem as do regular washings of the infected areas with cleavers tea. Washes can also be used on wounds and abscesses. Internal treatment can be used for epilepsy, anemia, dropsy, nervous complaints and constriction of the vocal cords. Toms suffering from a blocked bladder will be greatly helped by a regular dose of cleavers as the tea dissolves gravely deposits in the bladder. Cancer of the tongue and mouth and other cancerous growths are helped.

Coltsfoot

Actions - Expectorant, anti-spasmodic, demulcent, anti-catarrhal, diuretic.

The Latin name means banish cough.. Coltsfoot combines a soothing expectorant action with a anti spasmodic action. There are useful zinc levels in this plant. Consider this herb in any respiratory problem.

Uses - Coughs, pneumonia, asthma, pleurisy, TB, sedative powers in epilepsy, chronic or acute bronchitis, emphysema, cystitis.

Externally - A poultice is used for abscess, ulcers, boils, earache and toothache.

Cats and Dogs - Most particularly a chest herb with powerful expectorant and anti-inflammatory properties. Excellent for cases of bronchitis, bronchial asthma, pleurisy, Feline Respiratory Disease and chest problems that accompany a range of feline fungal diseases. It can be given with honey and lemon when coughing is a persistent problem. Can be used as a poultice for non-healing wounds. Ear infections can be helped by the fresh juice.

Comfrey

Actions - Demulcent, Astringent, Expectorant, Vulnerary.

Once widely cultivated as a fodder plant, sheep and cows eat it greedily, the impressive wound healing powers of comfrey are partially due to allantoin which stimulates cell proliferation and speeds the healing process inside and out.

Uses - Its old name is knit bone and that describes well what it does. Comfrey also guards against scar tissue from developing incorrectly, all internal hemorrhages including uterine, reunion of wound and fractures, internal ulcers, ruptures, pulmonary problems, bronchitis, irritable cough, ulcerative colitis, skin ulcers and varicose veins.

Cats and Dogs - One of the best wound and bone setting herbs. The tincture is effective of curing rheumatism and swollen joints even where arthritis has caused extensive damage. The tincture has been used for paralysis. Massage well into the joints and muscles of the affected parts. Where paralysis is due to shock, dislocation or sprain apply as a poultice. A cold infused tisane prepared overnight from the roots is good for digestive ailments, bronchitis, internal bleeding in the stomach, lungs or bowels, pleurisy and internal ulcers.

Corn Silk

Actions - Diuretic, demulcent, tonic, cystitis, prostrate.
A soothing diuretic that is helpful in any irritation of the membranes of the urinary system. Combined with other herbs in the treatment of cystitis, urethritis and prostatitis. Cleanses and soothes the urinary system.
Cats and Dogs - Good for the treatment of obesity and as it is a powerful diuretic it can be used for all complaints of the bladder and kidneys especially stones, edema, fluid in the heart, nephritis, cystitis, renal colic, and rheumatism.

Dandelion

Actions - Diuretic, cholagogue, anti-rheumatic, laxative, tonic.
The herb is blood cleansing and tonic, it has an important effect on the hepatic system and is a supreme jaundice curative herb, the leaves strengthen the enamel of the teeth and the white   juices of the freshly crushed stem dissolves warts, the plant is well grazed by goats, horses will take quantities of the leaves when cut and well mixed with bran, excellent for anemia because it is high in iron, calcium, copper

and vitamins, useful in kidney and bladder problems, skin eruptions, sluggish blood flow, weak arteries, all liver complaints, jaundice, constipation, gallbladder problems and rheumatism.

Cats and Dogs - A good liver herb especially for gall bladder complaints. It can be used for eczema and feline miliary dermatitis and is a healing tonic for the spleen. Internal digestive toning and cleansing along with metabolic disorders.

Elder

Actions - Expectorant, diaphoretic, flu, hay fever, sinusitis, purgative, flowers are anti-catarrhal.

Most animals will graze on elder. Used for the treatment of all gastric, hepatic, and pulmonary ailment, all fevers, skin disorders especially scabies and ring worm, externally as an insecticide. Elder is mainly used to treat colds, flu, dry coughs, sinusitis and catarrh.

Feverfew

Actions - Anti-inflammatory, vasodilator, relaxant, digestive bitter, uterine stimulant.

It is one of the most important aids for female ailments the plant exerting remarkable powers over the uterus, the whole plant is used. Has a good reputation for headaches, may help with arthritis when it is in the inflammatory stage. Digestive aid and tonic, inflamed or weak uterus and uterine and vaginal ulcers, abortion, difficult labor, retained afterbirth, arthritis, inflammations.

Fenugreek

Actions - Expectorant, demulcent tonic, galactagogue, lymphatic drainage.

The plant possesses highly aromatic seeds having a powerful disinfectant and emollient lubricant properties. The feeding value of these is about equal to linseed. It is one of the great fattening herbs. The perfect sister herb for garlic enhancing all its powers. Very tonic and eagerly sought by all animals. Rich in vitamins and nitrates, calcium and phosphorus. The whole plant is used. Good for all gastric weaknesses and ailments, nerves and neuralgia, female ailments including failing milk supply, allergies, bronchitis, anemia, bruises, colitis, coughs, diabetes, fever, flu, hay fever, headache, migraines, lung problems, sinus congestion, ulcers, reduces inflammation.

Ginger

Actions - Carminative, diaphoretic, circulatory stimulant, anti-inflammatory.

Ginger is warming and disinfectant and contains many healing virtues. Has a good action on the circulatory system and inflammations of the joints. Can be added to a formula to force assimilation and good for travel sickness.

Garlic

Actions - Anti-septic, anti-viral, diaphoretic, cholagogue, anti-spasmodic, hypotensive.

The plant is rich in volatile oil and sulphur and because of its remarkable penetrating, disinfecting and mucous expelling powers garlic is a valuable basic remedy for the treatment of all ailments in which the cleansing of the blood stream and expulsion of mucous accumulations is required. Garlic is extremely effective in dissolving and cleansing cholesterol from the blood stream, it stimulates the digestive tract, kills worms, parasites and harmful bacteria, normalizes blood pressure, reduces fever, gas and cramps. Use for all infections, coughs, colds, flu, bronchitis, all fevers, pulmonary conditions, gastric and skin complaints, rheumatism, all worms and also liver fluke, mange, ringworm, ticks and lice.

Caution - There is a lot of contradictory information out there about garlic for dogs saying it causes anemia. Sort term use would be alright.

Golden Rod

Actions - Anti-inflammatory, antiseptic, diaphoretic, flu, anti-catarrhal, cystitis, diaphoretic, carminative, diuretic, astringent, tonic, hypotensive.

It is famed as a wound herb, is a important remedy for female disorders, all cattle eat it and it brings them into good appetite and gives bloom, the whole plant is used, traditionally used for inflammation, upper respiratory catarrh, use with other herbs for influenza, flatulent dyspepsia, as a urinary anti-inflammatory and anti-septic, cystitis, urethritis and also used for urinary stones. This herb is also used for arthritis.

Uses - A powerful digestive aid, treatment of jaundice, kidney problems.

Externally - For wounds, to stop bleeding, cleansing gangrenous conditions.

Cat and Dog - The blossoms are gathered to treat intestinal ulceration and bleeding of the intestines as well as dysentery, vomiting and flatulence. Leaves and flowers are used for kidney complaints as well as urinary and bladder problems.

Dosage of infusion - Give a cat 1/2 teaspoon orally or in food 2 x daily.
Double the amount for dogs.

Horehound

Actions - Expectorant, antispasmodic, bitter.
Is one of the most important pectoral herbs a famed cough and throat remedy, the bitter action stimulates the flow of bile and thus improves digestion. Use for the treatment of cough, pneumonia, pleurisy, bronchitis, atrophy of the lungs, ear disorders, diarrhea, inflammation of the liver, jaundice.

Horsetail

Actions - Astringent, diuretic, enlarged prostate, incontinence.

Goats eat the plant but it is not a good food for cows, excellent astringent for the genito-urinary system reducing bleeding and healing wounds thanks to its high silica content, inflammation of the prostrate, tones and astringes the urinary system making it a good remedy for incontinence and bed wetting. Use for kidney stones as the high silica content erodes stones. May speed up the healing of bone, flesh and cartilage due to its high mineral content.

Uses - Nasal hemorrhage, laryngitis, intestinal ulcer, inflammation of the uterus, vagina and bladder, dysentery, enlarged anal glands, obesity, dropsy, a strong dose dissolves stones in the bladder.

Caution - If used over a long period it may decrease vitamin B1.

Cats and Dogs - Good for stopping internal bleeding and vomiting of blood. Used for kidney and bladder problems, gravel and stones.

Hyssop

Actions - Expectorant, antispasmodic, sedative, carminative, diaphoretic.

An important plant in pectoral complaints because it removes mucous accumulations and also tones up the membranes and fortifies the whole system. Is a mild vermifuge the Nordic countries use it as a vermifuge for delicate lambs and kids. Coughs, bronchitis, chronic catarrh, colds and flu's, anxiety states, hysteria, petit mal. Use for the treatment of cough, sore throat, pneumonia, pleurisy, worms, eye disorders, conjunctivitis.

Ladys Mantle

Actions - Astringent, emmenagogue, anti-inflammatory, diuretic.

This herb has a affinity to the womb where it helps with pain, bleeding and getting the cycle back to normal. Horses, goats and sheep seek out the herb, the plant is tonic and an important fortifier for the blood and walls of the arteries, it is a old herbal remedy for diabetes, reduces period pains and excessive bleeding, diarrhea, sores, ulcers a good menopause herb.

Uses - Treatment for lack of appetite, wasting, weak blood, sluggish blood, all weaknesses of the arteries, heart disease, taken from one period to another it is reputed to aid conception in barren animals.

Cats and Dogs - A good female herb for abdominal ailments, injuries after delivery or damage and debility, to strengthen the developing foetus in the womb, for inclination to miscarry and prolapse of the uterus.

Licorice

Actions - Demulcent, laxative, adrenal stimulant,

expectorant, sialagogue.

The root part is used , possessing unique pectoral and emollient properties, it is also nutritive and slightly laxative, It contains the building blocks of hormones, has a marked effect on the endocrine system, catarrh, bronchitis, coughs, gastric and peptic ulcers, abdominal colic. Use for the treatment of cough, inflamed throat, pneumonia, pleurisy, all catarrhal conditions, gallstones, chronic constipation, mild worms in young animals, female infertility, pains of colic.

Marshmallow

Actions - Demulcent, diuretic, emollient, vulnerary.

The foliage of the mallow is eaten by all animals, the roots are the main part used in internal medicine and also the leaves which are especially used for inflammation of the stomach and bowel, it contains over half its weight in sweet tasting mucilage which possess unique properties of lubricating, soothing and healing. A poultice can be used for all inflammatory conditions. Use for the treatment of sore throats, pulmonary catarrhs, pleurisy, diarrhea, dysentery, bowel inflammations and hemorrhages.

Meadowsweet

Actions - Acid balancer, stomachic, anti-inflammatory, astringent, pain killer.

A important fever and diarrhea herb, the gypsies use as a spring tonic for their animals, eaten plentifully by goats and sheep, acts to protect and soothe the mucous membranes of the digestive tract reducing excess acidity and easing nausea, heart burn, hyperacidity, gastritis, peptic ulcers. Not for Cats as they don't like the Aspirin part of this herb.

Mistletoe

Actions - Nervine, hypotensive, cardiac depressant, nervous tachycardia.

A tea is given in cases of chronic cramps, frostbite, hardening of the arteries, stroke, bleeding of the lungs and intestines, disorders of the uterus especially bleeding, is good as a general blood stauncher.

Nettles

Actions - Astringent, tonic, diuretic.

Used to treat rheumatism, arthritis, defective circulation and it also can relieve depression, bronchitis and reduces the risk of hemorrhage. It is perhaps the best blood herb which it purifies and renews. It cleanses the stomach and circulatory system ridding the body of eczema and other chronic skin disorders. Tonic for the pancreas and cleans the urinary system.

Parsley

Actions - Diuretic, carminative, emmenagogue, expectorant.

Well-liked by sheep and goats, improves their milk

yield and keeps them free from foot ills. It is a great enricher of the blood being very rich in iron and copper. Nutrient, digestive tract tonic, diuretic, high in potassium minerals and vitamins, bladder and kidney infections, incontinence, blood cleanser, immune builder, tonic for the blood vessels, aids in afterbirth pains, mainly used as a diuretic, carminative and emmenagogue. Good for the treatment of all disorders of the kidneys and bladder, gravel, stones, congestion, cystitis, jaundice, obesity, dropsy, worms, rheumatism, sciatica, swellings of the joints, the root can be used for constipation and obstructions of the intestines.

For any Animals that are recovering from an illness, surgery or toxic kidney problems.

Dogs: - Use larger amounts of parsley tea – 1- 2 tablespoon 3/4 times daily.

Can also add finely chopped parsley into their daily meals once or twice a week to help keep kidneys cleansed and free of disease.

Plantain

Actions - Expectorant, demulcent, astringent, diuretic.

Goats and sheep enjoy its foliage and poultry seek out the seeds. Plantain clears heat and removes excess fluid from the body while at the same time soothing inflammation and irritated tissues. The whole plant yields soothing mucilage similar to linseed, gentle expectorant while soothing sore and inflamed membranes, coughs, bronchitis etc. Its astringency aids in diarrhea and cystitis where there is bleeding. Is good for using in the treatment of stomach ulcers and has been used for blood poisoning. The plant is high in chlorophyll and good for use on wounds.

Uses - Treatment of dysentery, hemorrhages, internal obstructions and ulcers, fevers.

Externally - Wounds, sores, ulcers and all bites, eye disorders.

Cats and Dogs - Plantain is used for the entire range of diseases of the respiratory organs, particularly congested lungs, bronchial asthma and TB. It purifies the blood, lungs and stomach and is good for bad blood, kidney disorders, eczema, herpes and coughs. It helps convalescents especially when they need to gain weight. Also used in liver and bladder diseases.

Rosemary

Actions - Circulatory and nerve stimulant, carminative, antispasmodic, anti-depressive.

The powdered form is used on wounds as a antiseptic, nerve tonic, carminative, insecticide, acts as a circulatory and nerve stimulant, headache. Used in the treatment of all ailments of the heart, rheumatism, fits, epilepsy, paralysis, gastritis, diarrhea, dysentery.

Sage

Actions - Carminative, antispasmodic, astringent,

antiseptic.

Sage is well liked by animals and as with other aromatics makes the milk refreshing, tonic and increases the milk yield, it is a nervine, digestive and blood cleanser, a first rate remedy for all disorders of the throat, lungs and ears, inflamed and bleeding gums, inflamed tongue or general mouth inflammation, mouth ulcers, a good mouth wash.

Uses - Treatment of nerve debility, paralysis, all gastric ailments, constipation, obesity and female ailments, eczema, fevers, wound infections.

Caution - Stimulates the muscles of the uterus so should be avoided during pregnancy.

Cats and Dogs - For inflammations of the mouth, throat and tonsils.

Shepherds Purse

Actions - Uterine stimulant, astringent, diuretic.

Possesses important astringent properties, all animals like this herb and poultry seek it eagerly. A gentle diuretic, diarrhea, wounds, reduces excessive menstruation.

Uses - Treatment of hemorrhages internal and external, profuse bleeding of deep wounds, kidney ailments, female problems.

Cats and Dogs - For all internal and external bleeding tisanes should be given, helpful in muscular complaints and muscular atrophy.

Slippery Elm

Actions - Demulcent, astringent, nutrient.

Slippery elm bark provides a nutritious gruel which also possesses remarkable medicinal properties acting as a poultice both internally and externally. A nutrient and food for very old or young or weak cats and dogs, coats and heals all inflamed tissues internally and externally and is used for the stomach, intestines, ulcers, ulcerative colitis, enteritis, dysentery, constipation, internal bleeding of the digestive tract. Use for treatment of all digestive complaints especially ulcers for which it is a specific, dysentery, all pectoral disorders including TB, lung and bronchial hemorrhage, wasting diseases, rickets, stunted growth.

Speedwell

Actions - Expectorant, diuretic, stomachic, tonic.

Has a strong purifying action and will clear bronchitis, digestive disorders and asthma. It is also effective in the treatment of sores, eczema and ulcers especially when they are of the moist weeping kind. It rids the intestines of mucous and unhealthy deposits and can also be used for liver and spleen disorders.

St Johns Wort

Actions - Anti-inflammatory, astringent, sedative, nervine, anti-viral, nerve pains, anti-spasmodic, vulnerary, antibacterial.

The name St Johns Wort came from the Knights of St John of Jerusalem who used the herb to treat battle wounds.

Uses - Taken internally has a sedative and pain reducing effect, neuralgic pain, anxiety, tension, rheumatic pain, sciatica, for pains that shoot along the nerves, as a lotion it will speed the healing of wounds and bruises and is used where there is damage to the nerve rich areas, varicose veins and mild burns. Good for inflamed joints and rheumatic pain. In humans recently the herb has become popular to use as a antidepressant especially for cases of anxiety. Use as a lotion on wounds especially in the nerve rich areas such as the lips and fingers. As a lotion it is commonly mixed with Calendula, Homoeopaths call this lotion Hypercal.

Caution - Animals that overdose on Hypericum especially cattle become photosensitive and have to be locked in the barn for a while so as not to become sun burnt.

Cats and Dogs - Excellent wound herb and good for all nerve injuries. Good for highly strung, hysterical cats and dogs or those who have suffered some emotional or physical trauma.

Thyme

Actions - Carminative, antimicrobial, antispasmodic, astringent, expectorant, anthelmintic.

Used for laryngitis, sore throat and tonsils as well as being good for digestive infections and problems.

Valerian

Actions - Sedative, antispasmodic, carminative, anxiety, anti-depressive, hypotensive.

A powerful nervine and sedative stronger than other herbal sedatives, pain reliever, reduces anxiety, hysteria, sooths the nervous system, reduces high blood pressure, slows and strengthens the heart and calms palpitations, useful for muscle spasm, arthritic pain, spinal injuries, aids indigestion and gas, insomnia, cramps, colic, can help with migraines. Used for the treatment of epilepsy, hysteria, acute constipation, worms, malaria, pain, sensitive nervous animals.

Yarrow

Actions - Diuretic, antiseptic, diaphoretic, peripheral vaso dilator, hypotensive, bitter tonic.

All abdominal complaints even cancer. When the queen suffers from inflammation of the ovaries or prolapse of the uterus, for feline respiratory disease to relieve congestion and running eyes. Bone marrow problems and diseases, bleeding from the lungs and stomach, good for flatulence , indigestion and abdominal cramps, soothes the gastro intestinal tract and calms diarrhea. Gives the kidneys a boost. Good for fevers.

Witch Hazel

Actions - Astringent one of the most widely used ones. Antiseptic.

As with all astringents this herb may be used where ever there is bleeding both externally and internally, commonly used for piles, bruises and inflamed swellings, varicose veins, diarrhea. Use internally to heal ulcerated and burnt tissues in cases of poisoning, stomach and intestinal ulcers, Externally - wounds, sores, bruises, ulcers, inflammation of the organs of reproduction, torn udders resulting in milk leakage, inflamed udders and glands, sore eyes and inflamed ears.

Homeopathic Supplement

Homeopathy has been around now for hundreds of years and unlike most other forms of medicine its rules have not changed and will not for they are based on a essential truth. The main rule is Like cures Like or if we break down the word Homeopathy homo means the same and pathy means disease. As Homoeopathy is a very hard science to learn and as it kind of sits or balances on the border of hard science and metaphysics I will not try to explain to you what it is here as it would probably take a whole book to do this but I will say this, in the UK and a lot of countries in Europe it is on and paid for by the National Health System and anything that can get a politician to open their purse must work.

It is said that Homeopathy sits on a three legged stool. What this means is that if a remedy has at least three symptoms in the same strength as the symptoms you are trying to match then that remedy is a potential cure for your condition or if not cure it will offer the condition relief. The more symptoms you can match to the remedy the better the remedy will work for the rule is likes cure likes not vaguely similar cures. Listed below are some common Homoeopathic Remedies and some of the symptoms they cover. The idea is to find one remedy that covers most of your symptoms. To make the remedies as closer a match as we can we ask lots of questions like the ones below and after we gather all the answers we have what is called a good Symptom Picture which we then try to match as accurately as we can to a Remedy. Most Homeopathic Materia Medicas are set out to answer the questions listed below with the mind symptoms being the most important. Questions on time, position and temperature are good for making a choice between to very close remedies. The best Materia Medica for the lay person is Boerickes and you should be able to view this on a few Homeopathic websites.

Symptom Guide Questions

1/. Was there a sudden onset of the condition, at what time?

2/. What time of the day does the patient feel either better or worse.

3/. What is the effect of motion? jarring? walking? running?

4/. What is the effect of drinking fluids? warm and or cold drinks?

5/. Is the patient thirsty or not at all? sips or gulps?

6/. Is the onset from exertion? overeating? weather changes? emotions?

7/. Mental emotional state of patient?

8/. Better warm room? warm air?

9/. Better cool room? cool open air?

10/. Are the respirations upper chest movements or in the abdomen?

11/. Respirations - dry or wet?

12/. Expectoration - watery or stringy mucous, easy or

difficult.

13/. Is there coughing

14/. Position - better or worse from sitting? standing? lying? lying on which side?

15/. Along with the condition is there fever? gas? belching? wind?

Modality - The questions above are covering what the Homoeopaths call modalities which basically mean are covering a condition that makes the patient better or worse. I will list the main Modalities below. The Modalities help us to distinguish which remedy is right for the case especially when we have a group that look as though they may all work which is what I am giving you und the disease heading. Using modalities forces you to think what really is going on, is this the nature of the beast or the nature of the disease.

Time - Better or Worse morning, night, weekly, monthly, seasonally etc.

Motion - Better or Worse first movement, rest, exertion, walking, stretching, rising up etc

Temperature - Better or Worse heat, cold, cold air blowing, sudden change etc.

Body Activity - Better or Worse eating, drinking, urinating, defecating, sleep, coughing etc

Weather - - Better or Worse, damp, sunny, foggy, storms, sudden changes etc.

Senses - Better or Worse - touch, pressure, noise, light, odors etc.

Position - Better or Worse lying, standing, sitting, stretched out, doubled up, right side etc.

Mind - Excitement, anger, fear, stress, better busy, nervous all the time etc.

Now read through all the remedies in the Marteria Medica (Homoeopathic Remedy Reference) and you will notice that most of them have Mind or mental symptoms kind of describing the personalities or moods a good example is Nux Vomica, I think we all know a nasty type of individual that this remedy would be suited to and meaning as though the individual is suited to this remedy then the remedy would have a curative action on them but don't expect it to change the nature of the beast. One of the main rules of Homeopathy is the closer the match of the remedy the higher the Potency you use but if you are not used to Homoeopathy just use the 30C potency and remember what I said about the 3 legged stool. Potency is a measure of strength and depth of action.

Remember as mentioned before Homoeopathy sits on a three legged stool. What this means is that if a remedy has at least three symptoms in the same strength as your symptoms then that remedy is a potential cure.

Note - The best prescribing guide for the layman is **Boerickes Materia Medica With Repertory.**

Another good guide is **The Complete Book Of Homeopathy by Dr Michael Weiner.**

I always buy my books on Homeopathy from India as

they are quarter the price and there is always a wide selection. Put B. Jain Publishers into the google search engine go to their web site and check out these books and I am sure you will be pleased with what you find.

Disease Nosodes

Nosodes are remedies made from disease material mainly from the tissues, discharges, exudates, excretions, suppurations or secretions of a infected being. Simply stated a Nosode is a homeopathic remedy prepared from a pathological specimen. Rabies Nosode, for example starts with the saliva of a rabid dog and is then potentized.

Nosodes have many uses and are widely used in homeopathic practice to help limit cases of infectious diseases and to help during the recovery phase of a disease especially the ones that linger and drag on. There are Nosodes for most infectious diseases of animals and humans the use of Nosodes in this way is referred to as isopathy rather than Homoeopathy. They are often used in farm situations, to limit the spread and the effects of infectious diseases. This has especially been used as a vital component of mastitis control on many farms, both organic and conventional. One documented event about Nosodes dates back to Napoleon marching his Legions through Europe and spreading Typhoid in their wake, the towns that had the best cure rates were the ones where the local Homoeopaths used a Nosode of the disease.

Nosodes can be used in the prevention of infectious diseases in the manner of vaccination but they work by a completely different mechanism then from the raising of antibodies that vaccines work by. As yet it is not actually known how they work but they have survived hundreds of years ridicule by producing results and will carry on doing so.

The best known study into Nosodes was done by Dr. Christopher Day of England involving 'kennel cough' in a boarding kennel. At the time he was called in, there were 40 dogs in the kennel with 35 that had kennel cough. About half had been vaccinated for this malady. He gave a Nosode to all the animals that were there and all the dogs that came in through the rest of the summer, which was another 214 dogs. He successfully reduced the incidence of kennel cough from over 90% to less than 2%.

Nosodes used for the prevention of diseases are usually given in the 30C potency. A good dosing regime is one dose given night and morning for 3 days followed by one per month for the next 6 months. This generally provides a good level of protection after the first week. A good example of how this can be used is a puppy given the Nosode of Parvovirus at 3 to 4 weeks of age instead of having to wait for 9 weeks for the vaccination, this way the puppy is protected before given the vaccination.

Nosodes can have homeopathic therapeutic properties in their own right. Such Nosodes are found in the Homoeopathic Materia Medica and have undergone a proper 'proving'. Examples are

Bacillinum, Carcinosinum, Medorrhinum, Psorinum, Tuberculinum.

Dose - Dr. Surjit S. Makker recommends 20ml of remedy mixed with 8 liters of water for 100 birds. This medicated water should be shaken well and put in drinkers accordingly. For individual birds give them 2-3 pellets by mouth and keep them calm.

Notes

Materia Medica

Note - All Homeopathic Remedies are given in Potency and not in material Form.

Aconite

Characteristics - Aconite is best used in the first stages of a illness, especially when fear and anxiety are present. Symptoms appear suddenly, without warning and they may be caused by exposure to cold winds or draughts or by a severe fright. Symptoms are a marked restlessness, animal displays extreme anxiety or fear, high fever with a burning skin, extreme sweating and a burning thirst, a hoarse dry painful cough, bright light noises stress and cold worsen the symptoms, rest and quiet relieves the symptoms. The pains of Aconite are unbearable, sharp, shooting, burning pains, tingling and numbness. A remedy for fevers and inflammatory states, use at the first sign of all fevers, shivering with cold sweats, difficult breathing, animal shows desire for large quantities of water, symptoms worse at midnight, symptoms improve in the open air.

Mind - Great fear, anxiety, restlessness, extreme sensitivity to pain, worry, foreboding.

Better - In open air, warmth, rest.

Worse - In the evening and night, particularly before midnight, lying on affected side.

Allium Cepa

Characteristics - Increased secretions from the eyes and nose, like those of the common cold. Frequent sneezing with watery discharge which burns the nose and upper lip, but the eye discharge is bland and doesn't burn (the opposite of Euphrasia). Tickling in the throat with incessant cough (feels as if larynx is split) holds throat when coughing. Being in cool open air relieves the symptoms, eyelids are swollen and red, abdominal tympany with wind, this remedy is indicated in the early stages of most catarrhal conditions, mild forms of cat flu can be cut short if given early.

Better - Cold room (except cough), open air.

Worse - Evening, warm room, odors.

Antimonium Tartaricum - Ant Tart

Characteristics - Is characterized by a loose rattling unproductive cough such as is often herd in cats. Respiration can be very difficult with much gasping. There is usually thirst for little and often. Symptoms are worse in the evening, lying down and in cold damp weather or a warm room. Confined largely to respiratory diseases, abundant bronchial secretions, great rattling of mucous with little expectoration, drowsiness, debility and sweat.

Mind - Drowsy and despondent, fear of being alone, child will not be touched without whining.

Better - Sitting erect, from burping and

expectoration.

Worse - Evenings, lying down, damp cold weather.

Apis

Characteristics - Apis is used for various types of swelling and inflammation such as that from animal bites and bites and stings from insects, it is also used for measles, mumps, sore throats, sore red eyes and fever. Apis is a quick acting remedy for inflammations especially those ones with edema and lots of swelling which is its main use. Acute nephritis with scanty and burning urine there may be some blood in the urine. . Symptoms are swelling with edema which makes the effected parts look shiny, red and puffy, the swollen parts feel soggy and waterlogged, a fever that develops rapidly but without thirst, extreme restlessness and fidgeting, an irritable nature and perhaps jealous, cool air and cold compresses relieve the symptoms. Pains are burning and stinging, arthritis with swelling, animals seek cold surface to lie on, swollen eyelids, may be swollen ears, may be blood in the urine, in the horse and cow there may be edema in the lower limbs while in dogs abdominal dropsy is seen. Symptoms get worse from heat and improve in the open air and from cold bathing.

Mind - Apathy, indifference, awkward.

Better - By cold, (room, air or application)

Worse - From warmth, pressure, late in the

afternoon, from sleeping.

Arnica

Characteristics - Bruises and similar injuries where the skin is unbroken and there is mental or emotional shock. Symptoms are any type of bruising or similar injury caused by crushing, squeezing or wrenching, muscles strains which feel sore and bruised, shock after accidents, there is a fear of being touched because of the pain, good for the soreness after birth and medical operations.

Arnica can be used in potency and also as a cream. The cream must not be used on broken skin or wounds. Animal shrinks away when you try to touch it, symptoms improve when lying down.

Mind - Fears touch or approach, whole body oversensitive.

Better - Lying down or with head low.

Worse - Least touch, motion, damp and cold.

Arsenic Album

Characteristics - Burning pains relieved by heat, anxious, restless, weak and chilly with an air of fear and hopelessness. Anxiety or restlessness are often present where this remedy is indicated. Discharge from eyes and nose are watery and acrid causing ulceration in those regions. The mouth is usually dry and the patient is usually thirsty. Dramatic vomiting and diarrhea often simultaneously indicate its use if the modalities agree. The patient may have wheezing respiration and allergic asthmatic conditions can respond well. The skin can be dry, scaly and scruffy. Symptoms are worse for cold and wet better for warmth. Tries to find relief in motion but immediately feels weak with movement. Restless, feels cold, complains of general weakness, discharges burn the skin.

Mind - Fear with despair and restlessness.

Better - Warmth, open air, relieved by sweat, hot drinks, lying down (but restless).

Worse - Cold air, after midnight eg 1 to 3am. Wet damp weather and near sea shore.

Belladonna

Characteristics - This is one of the great fever remedies, conditions requiring its use usually being of violent and sudden onset. Heat, redness, pain and swelling characterize its symptoms. It is one of the main remedies used in convulsions. Pupils are usually dilated which is a keynote for this remedy. Acute ear inflammation where there is heat, pain and swelling respond well. The mouth is usually dry and there is great thirst. With Belladonna always think BIRDS. B for burning, I for irritability, R for redness, D for delirium and S for spasms.

Mind - Hallucinations, delirium, rages, bites, strikes, desire to escape.

Better - For quiet, dark, rest with slight warmth.

Worse - For noise, touch or jarring motion.

Bellis Perennis

Characteristics - Trauma to abdomen and pelvic organs especially after surgery and child birth if arnica does not give relief. Injuries to the nerves with intense soreness, back ache from hard physical work such as gardening, pain is bruised sore and aching, better cold presses, worse touch, after getting wet.

The animal is unwilling to move and when made to do so evinces pain, muscular stiffness is prominent.

Worse - Left side and cold wind.

Bryonia

Characteristics - This remedy shows both diarrhea and constipation symptoms, the latter usually in chronic conditions. The mouth is often dry and there is great thirst. The tongue is often coated yellow. It is of great help in many cases of rheumatism or arthritis where the symptoms agree. There is often respiratory signs with a hoarse hacking cough. All symptoms are worse for movement and better for rest.

Mind - Irritable, delirium.

Better - Lying on the painful side, pressure, rest and cold things.

Worse - Warmth, motion, morning, eating and touch.

Calendula

Characteristics - The part used is the Flowers and it is used for wounds and skin irritations, it is healing, soothing, anti-inflammatory, astringent, anti-fungal and anti-microbial.

Use as a lotion for cuts, grazes, infected sores, fungal infections, any skin inflammations, regulates the oil production of the skin so is good for acne, to stop bleeding, for bruises and sprains, skin ulcers and minor burns and scolds.

Note - The tincture of this is used as a lotion diluted at 1 to 10.

Cantharis

Characteristics - Important first aid remedy for minor burns and for other pains that feel burning and fiery, also has a healing effect on the bladder, urethra and other parts of the urinary tract where burning pain is the key symptom, burns and scalds especially where blistering and inflammation occur, sunburn, insect bites that feel hot and burn, cystitis. Pains are violent burning, cutting, stabbing or smarting, rawness, use when the animal appears distressed when passing urine, or tries to pass and cannot. Better from warmth rest and rubbing.

Mind - Furious delirium, acute mania generally of a sexual type, crying, barking.

Better - From rubbing

Worse - From touch or approach, from urinating,

from drinking cold water.

Carbo Vegetabilis

Characteristics - Patient exhibits mental and physical sluggishness and symptoms come on slowly, generalized weakness of all functions especially digestion, overweight, torpid, lazy, complaints of coldness, pains usually described as burning, pressing pains, wishes to be fanned, digestive problems such as belching often accompany any illness.

Mind - Aversion to darkness, sudden loss of memory.

Better - Being fanned, passing gas, rest.

Worse - Morning and evening, exertion, cold, tight clothes at abdomen.

Causticum

Characteristics - Burns and burning pains such as cystitis also used for dry coughs, burns to the skin especially with marked inflammation and blistering, coughs, laryngitis and hoarseness from straining and over using voice, cystitis especially with involuntary passing of urine when coughing, chronic cystitis, exposure to cold dry air may make symptoms worse.

Mind - Least thing makes it cry, sad, hopeless. Ailments from long lasting grief.

Better - In damp wet weather, warmth.

Worse - Cold winds.

Euphrasia

Characteristics - Affects the mucous membranes of the eyes, nose and chest producing copious watery secretions,eye secretions cause smarting of the skin while the nose discharge is bland. Used for conjunctivitis, eye strain generally but especially from computers, eyes that feel sore and inflamed and look red, hay fever symptoms including a tickly throat, sneezing, a runny nose, and itchy red watering eyes. Sunlight wind and warmth worsen the symptoms. Use for Dogs who have had their head out of the window for to long, symptoms better in dim light or darkness, in all species a tendency to diarrhea occurs.

Better - In the dark

Worse - From light, indoors, in the evening.

Hypericum

Characteristics - Used for bruises and other injuries especially to nerve rich areas like the fingers, lips, ears, eyes ,tail bone, good for the pain of puncture wounds of any cause e.g. animal or insect. Helps with the pains after operations especially amputations. Pains are violent shooting pains along a nerve path, burning, tingling and numbness. Worse from shock and touch and better from rubbing, horse fly bites, symptoms worse cold better warmth.

Mind - Anxiety, melancholy, effects of shock.

Better - Bending head backward.

Worse - Cold, dampness and touch.

Ipecac

Characteristics - Indicated for complaints of persistent nausea not relieved by vomiting, ailments caused by eating rich or indigestible type of foods such as ice-cream, sweets etc., useful to stop bleeding if blood is bright red.

Mind - Easily irritated, child cries or screams continuously, wanting something but not sure what they desire, holds everything in contempt.

Worse - Warm, moist weather, lying down.

Kali Bichromicum

Characteristics - Has a affinity for the mucous membranes of the body, tough stringy viscid secretions sometimes forming thick yellow green mucous, sinus infections, suited for fleshy fat light complexioned people, general weakness.

Better - Heat

Worse - Cold, beer, morning, undressing.

Kali Carbonicum

Characteristics - Has a affinity for the mucous membranes digestive and respiratory, very tired, anemic, flabby tissues which may be swollen, sweat, backache, weakness, many conditions have a aggravation at 2am to 4am, often stays immobile when ill.

Mind - Very irritable, hypersensitive to pain, despondent.

Better - During the day, sitting down, bending forward, warmth.

Worse - Cold weather, between 2am and 4am.

Lachesis

Characteristics - Many symptoms tend to be left sided, cannot bear tight clothing, symptoms worse on awakening, symptoms relieved with onset of the menstrual flow. Short dry cough, feels relief after coughing up watery phlegm, feeling of constriction in throat and chest, better bending forward.

Mind - Overly talkative, impatient, sad, jealous, no desire to mix with world.

Better - Release of pressure, eating fruit, cold, discharges.

Worse - Pressure, touch, after sleep, heat, hot weather.

Ledum

Characteristics - Has a action on the capillaries and is useful for cleaning up bruises especially around the eyes, mainly used for puncture wounds made by sharp points such as nails and wood splinters and insect bites and stings especially ones that don't heal properly and look blue and puffy. Wounds that feel cold to the touch, septic conditions, sprains, pains are throbbing, tearing ,prickling, they shoot upwards, stiff and sore. Better cold, cold bathing. This remedy was used in the past along with hypericum to ward off tetanus especially in deep wounds

Better - From cold.

Worse - At night and from heat.

Lycopodium

Characteristics - Exerts most of its effects on the digestive organs, liver, kidneys and respiratory systems. The patient dislikes being left alone and appears apprehensive. The nose is often blocked and there may be blisters on the tongue. Eating a little food always satisfies the appetite but appetite is very marked. The belly is usually bloated. The stool appears hard and small and is expelled only with difficulty accompanied by ineffectual straining. Urination is also a slow process and the urine has a red sediment. Symptoms are worse for heat generally and better for cold.

Mind - Melancholy, afraid to be alone, apprehensive.

Better - By motion, on getting cold.

Worse - From heat.

Natrum Sulphuricum

Characteristics - A good liver remedy, emotional and mental difficulties arising after head injury, useful in problems associated with rainy weather and dampness, patient feels every change from dry to wet weather, may remove excess water and fluid retention from the body.

Mind - Lively music saddens, melancholy, inability to think, dislikes to speak or be spoken to.

Better - Dry weather and environments, pressure, change of position.

Worse - Damp weather, damp basements, lying on left side.

Nux Vom

Characteristics - The remedy for overindulgence, adapted especially to thin irritable energetic people who attend with great detail to tasks, quarrelsome, nervous, intelligent, hypochondriacal, oversensitive to noise music and light, craves stimulants.

Primarily used in the digestive sphere, its greatest reputation is in helping disturbances following overeating of unsuitable foods. Feces is usually hard but diarrhea can follow overeating. There is abdominal discomfort, flatulence, irritability and sensitivity to noise. Symptoms are generally worse for noise and better after rest or for damp weather.

Mind - Very irritable, sensitive to all impressions, malicious, disposed to reproach others.

Better - Wet weather, lying down, uninterrupted nap.

Worse - Overeating, mental over exertion, sensory stimulation ie sound, sight, touch etc.

Phosphorus

Characteristics - Irritated and inflamed mucous and serous membranes are the key feature of this remedy. Is a very sudden remedy with suddenness of symptoms. The patient is sensitive to loud and sudden noises (eg thunder fireworks etc). Degenerative processes and bone destruction respond well to Phosphorus. Food is suddenly vomited back up when it has been warmed in the stomach, gums can be ulcerated and bloody. Hepatitis, jaundice, pancreatic disease and nephritis come into its sphere. Urine may be bloody. A very painful cough is also a symptom. Wounds that perpetually bleed may also be helped. The patient is usually in poor body condition. Symptoms are worse for touch, exertion, in the evening and during thunder storm. Better for cold and sleep.

Mind - Low spirits, restless, fidgety.

Better - In the dark, lying on the right side, from the cold, sleep.

Worse - Touch, from exertion and in the evening.

Pulsatilla

Characteristics - Often indicated for those with mild, gentle, timid yielding dispositions who are easily moved to laughter and tears, The Pulsatilla person wants to be held and loved, moods changeable and fickle, the patient is chilly but desires strolling in cold air, symptoms are erratic and change frequently, pains are wandering, pains that grow gradually in intensity, fever without thirst despite dry mouth, bland yellow discharges.

Mind - Weeps easily, timid, fears to be alone - dark - ghosts, likes sympathy and fuss, highly emotional, easily discouraged, sensitive.

Better - Open air, cold applications, consolation relieves symptoms.

Worse - Evening before midnight, warmth, after eating fat rich food.

Rhus Tox

Characteristics - Is the most famous of the rheumatic remedies. The skin and muscular skeletal system are its main spheres. Small red papules in the skin and sometimes vesicles are typical lesions with much scratching. In all cases of damage to muscles think of Rhus and the symptoms of arthritis which are worse after rest particularly if this follows strenuous exertion. The symptoms improve with limbering up , The worst pains are seen as the animal arises from its bed.

Mind - Listless, sad, extreme restlessness, great apprehension at night.

Better - Warmth, walking, from stretching out limbs.

Worse - During sleep, cold wet rainy weather and at night.

Ruta

Characteristics - Has effects on the joints, tendons, cartilages, and the periosteum which is a fine membrane that covers bones and gives it that shiny look, it is also used for eye strain where the vision goes dim.

Used for painful bruises affecting the bones, dislocations, strains to the tendons or joints, aching with restlessness, pains are gnawing, digging, burning, bruised, sore as if beaten, bones as if broken, pain deep in the bones, rheumatism.

Better - From lying and warmth.

Worse - From over exertion, touch, cold wet weather.

Silica

Characteristics - Fits the shy chilly patient who is reluctant to enter the room, chronic inflammatory conditions such as sinus, helps in the removal of foreign bodies such as splinters and seeds, ripens abscesses, ailments attended with pus formation. Use silica and be prepared to use it for a while sometimes up to 3 weeks.

Mind - Faint hearted, anxious, yielding.

Better - Warmth, wet or humid weather.

Worse - Morning, from lying down, cold.

Staphysagria

Characteristics - Suits sensitive people who suppress their feelings and suffer in silence or who boil over with indignation, remedy for cuts and wounds especially those that are from medical procedures and have the mentioned feelings. Nervous states of animals. The pains are stinging, stitching, smarting, squeezing, as if stabbed by a knife. Worse from touch, emotions and suppressed anger.

Better - Warmth, rest at night.

Worse - Touch on affected parts, loss of fluids.

Symphytum

Characteristics - Causes bone to grow and promotes fast healing should be given for all fractures. Used for injuries to the hard parts of the body while arnica is for the soft parts. Also used for eye injuries caused from blows.

Caution - do not use if a pin has been placed in the bone as the pin has to be removed latter.

Tarentula Cubensis

Characteristics - For abscesses, boils, carbuncles, swellings of any kind but especially on the back of the neck where the skin turns black, red/blue or purple with great pain. Deep septic conditions with hardening of the effected part, condition comes on fast, pains are burning, stinging, throbbing, pricking like a needle.

Worse - Night.

Urtica Urens

Characteristics - Can be used for burns and also for cystitis where the urine burns the skin and there is dificulty passing urine. Symptoms are stinging pains, swellings particularly blistery swellings, itching.

Worse - Cool moist air, touch.

Notes

Vitamin C

Vitamin C is the primary antioxidant in the lungs and a powerful antihistamine without side effects. Low vitamin C dramatically increases histamine levels which put you at greater risks for inflammation responses in the body. Always give a high dose of Vitamin C to animals before any operation where they require a anesthetic for the reasons mentioned above as they will recover faster and better from the anesthetic and maybe the inflammation from the surgical incisions will be toned down a bit.

Vitamin C is needed by the immune system and is necessary for healing and the prevention of infections along with being a potent antioxidant with anti-bacterial and antiviral actions. It is also essential for the utilization of the essential amino acids lysine (anti-viral) and proline. Another point to consider is that stress depletes the bodies supply of Vitamin C so this may be another factor in the cause of many diseases. Vit C is essential for the formation of collagen tissue which is vital in tendons and cartilage so always consider this in muscle and back injuries and especially trauma injuries.

Sodium Ascorbate is good for use on animals as it is virtually tasteless when added to the animal's food and does not curdle milk. This can be used in high doses when needed for example dose till the bowels become loose then back the dose off. For severe situations you can use a injectable Vitamin C, in Australia we use Troys Injectable Vit C which we get from the Agricultural Stock Feed Shops or Co Ops. Use a large gauge needle with this as some animals have rather thick hides and the liquid solution is also fairly thick.

Think of using Vitamin C in all operations and all acute diseases. It is a good last resort to think of before the rifle especially in the deadly acute diseases where as a last resort you would use the injectable form in a intramuscular injection, this can also be a good gauge as to what may happen as these injections hurt like hell so if the animal turns around and gives you a filthy look then there is a good chance that they may live and if they do not seem to notice the injection well the chances don't look too good. So remember always keep a bottle of Injectable C in the fridge for emergencies.

Good Herb Sources Of Vitamin C

Alfalfa, Burdock, Catnip, Cayenne, Chickweed, Dandelion, Hawthorn, Garlic, Horseradish, Kelp, Parsley, Plantain, Papaya, Raspberry, Rosehips, Shepherds Purse, Yellow Dock.

The Safest Essential Oils For Animal Use

Supplement To The Natural Remedies For Animal Series

Extreme care must be taken using the Essential Oils on animals. The ones mentioned in these pages seem to be the safest if used in a low dose which is a quarter of what you would use on a human and even this would be too high if used on a mouse so really think about what you are doing and always use a little test dose to check for sensitivity.

Danger - Do not use on **birds** and **cats** as there metabolism cannot handle Essential oils and death will be the most likely result, this includes Eucalyptus and Tea Tree oil.

How Oils Work

Essential Oils work by entering the blood stream via the pores of the skin so the biggest action is on the area applied followed by a systemic action via the blood. The liver is the main blood filter and detoxifier of the body so the liver is responsible for breaking down any drug or blood borne foreigner so with the Essential Oils there is always the chance that if the dose is too high or the application is to frequent the liver may be damaged. Never forget that oils are highly concentrated products. A good example is a budgie, you clipped the wings and one is now bleeding so you put Tea Tree oil on it. Imagine the size of one drop of oil now imagine the size of a Budgies liver and it's fairly obvious what's going to happen.

Below are given the cautions for using oils on dogs, follow these cautions on all animals in general. Most information for these pages was sourced from Kristen Leigh Bells book Holistic Aromatherapy For Animals and Catharine Birds book A Healthy Horse The Natural Way.

Essential Oil Blends

Soothing Skin Essential Oil Blend

15ml base oil of hazel nut or sweet almond oil

2 drops Geranium

6 drops Rosewood

6 drops Lavender

1 drop Roman Chamomile

2 drops Carrot Seed

Combine all ingredients, shake and store in a dark glass bottle. Use 2 to 4 drops of this blend to spot treat small areas of skin.

Mange Treatment Blend

15ml base oil of hazel nut or sweet almond oil

5 drops Lavender

7 drops Niaouli

1 drop Helichrysum

2 drops Sweet Marjoram

After bathing the dog 2 to 4 drops of the blend should be applied to the affected areas twice a day for at least

2 weeks. Observe for a week and repeat if necessary. Try to prevent the dog from licking the area.

Tick Bite Forula
15ml base oil of hazel nut or sweet almond oil
5 drops Thyme Thujanol
3 drops Hyssop Decumbens
8 drops Lavender
For use on bites or immediately after the tick is removed to help prevent infection, reduce redness and inflammation and possibly prevent Lymes disease.

Fresh Breath Oil Blend
5ml base oil of hazel nut or sweet almond oil
6 drops Cardamom
4 drops Coriander Seed
6 drops Peppermint
1 to 3 drops inside of the dogs mouth.

Calm Dog Blend
15ml base oil of hazel nut or sweet almond oil
3 drops Valerian
2 drops Vetiver
4 drops Petitgrain
3 drops Sweet Marjoram
2 drops Sweet Orange
The calming effect ranges from taking the edge off to soothing the dog. Dose is 1 to 6 drops depending on the size of the dog.

Fear or Seperation Anxiety

15ml base oil of hazel nut or sweet almond oil
1 drop Neroli
2 drops Sweet Bazil
4 drops Bergamot
6 drops Petitgrain
1 drop Ylang Ylang
Dose is 1 to 6 drops depending on size of dog.

Flea Free Blend

15ml base oil of hazel nut or sweet almond oil
4 drops Clary Sage
1 drop Citronella
7 drops Peppermint
3 drops Lemon
Store in dark glass bottle. 2 to 4 drops to the neck, chest, legs and tail base of the dog.

Tick Free Blend

15ml base oil of hazel nut or sweet almond oil
2 drops Geranium
2 drops Rosewood
3 drops Lavender
2 drops Myrhh
2 drops Opoponax
1 drop Bay Leaf
Store in dark glass bottle. 2 to 4 drops to the neck, chest, legs and tail base of the dog.

Increasing The Appetite

15ml base oil of hazel nut or sweet almond oil

2 drops Sweet Orange

2 drops Lemon

2 drops Grapefruit

2 drops Lime

2 drops Bergamot

For old and sick dogs this is a gentle appetite stimulant. 2 to 6 drops of the final blend to the neck and chest of the dog gently rubbed in. Repeat as needed up to 6 times per day.

Immune Boosting Blend

15ml base oil of hazel nut or sweet almond oil

2 drops Bay Laurel

2 drops Ravensare

2 drops Palmarosa

2 drops Eucalyptus

2 drops Niaouli

2 drops Coriander Seed

2 drops Thyme Thujanol

2 to 4 drops daily via massage to neck and chest.

Colds and Congestion

15ml base oil of hazel nut or sweet almond oil

5 drops Eucalyptus

5 drops Myrhh

5 drops Ravensare

For relieving nasal congestion or cold symptoms in dogs. 1 to 6 drops rubbed into neck or chest.

Fatigue Blend

15ml base oil of hazel nut or sweet almond oil

7 drops Rosemary
6 drops Tangerine
3 drops Ylang Ylang
Balancing and revitalizing for dogs that are suffering from fatigue and malaise.
2 to 4 drops daily via massage to neck and chest.

Flatulence Blend
15ml base oil of hazel nut or sweet almond oil
3 drops Caraway
3 drops Cardamom
3 drops Cinnamon
3 drops Nutmeg
3 drops Tangerine
1 to 2 drops placed on your dog's food and then 1 or 2 drops given after eating. Many dogs enjoy the taste of this spicy blend and will lick it off your hand. The spice oils of this blend are commonly found in food flavorings so digestion is regarded as safe.

Joint Rub Blend
15ml base oil of hazel nut or sweet almond oil
3 drops Black Pepper
4 drops Peppermint
3 drops Speramint
4 drops Juniper Berry
Good for muscle soreness, arthritis, hip dysplasia and sprains. use 2 to 4 drops of the blend and try to rub in as close to the skin as possible. Do a patch test with this oil as it can be irritating. Patch tests can be done with drop of blend in the arm pit.

Motion Sickness Blend
15ml base oil of hazel nut or sweet almond oil
7 drops Ginger
8 drops Peppermint
Give 3 drops in the mouth

Labor Ease Blend
15ml base oil of hazel nut or sweet almond oil
6 drops Clary Sage
1 drop Neroli
5 drops Petitgrain
2 drops Lavender
1 drop Roman Chamomile
Calming and balancing blend, can be applied to the fur of the neck or chest or 1 to 4 drops can be rubbed in the belly.

Oils For Horses

The safest way to use Essential Oils on your horse are external massage and inhalation. When inhaled the Oil addresses the horses emotional states and stored memories as well as entering the body and having an effect with the most obvious here being Eucalyptus which acts as a bronchodilator (illegal for competition horses in some parts of the US). **Use blends in the same strengths as mentioned in dogs don't go over 2% oil in a blend. Only apply the blends to the affected areas. You can copy** some of the dog formulas or make your own using the list of oils.

Essential Oils For Animal Use

The Essential Oils below are fairly safe for Animal Use

Basil (Sweet) - Helpful for restoring mental balance and clarity. For animals that are suffering nervousness or anxiety, dogs with separation anxiety. Use sparingly (PMC30%). **Horses** - Helps to release most muscle spasms. Used before a event it minimizes the amount of uric acid in the blood and other toxic wastes from exercise. A warming winter oil feeding the muscle fibers and stimulating the blood flow. It is a expectorant removing mucous from a clogged respiratory system when rubbed into the chest and inhaled. Rubbed into the abdomen it may help to relieve the pain and symptoms of colic. May irritate the skin in high doses and don't use in pregnancy.

Bay Leaf - Good for a hair and fur tonic, ticks don't like it, good deodorizer.

Actions - Ant microbial.

Bay Laurel - Used in blends for boosting the immune system especially in dogs. Use only in small amounts in blends.

Bergamot - Combines toning, strengthening and balancing effects with soothing, relaxing and uplifting qualities. Useful for the treatment of fungal conditions such as dog ear infections due to yeast overgrowth. Use in small doses as it can cause photosensitization. **Horse** - Use full for treating any skin complaint especially folliculitis, flaking skin and wounds. Good for lice infections and bites, aids in the healing of any wounds and reduces scar formation. Has a stimulating effect on appetite. Be cautious when applying to the skin of a gray horse or to sensitive skin areas that will be exposed to the sun as this oil can cause photosensitization or pigment changes.

Black Pepper - Warming and circulatory stimulant qualities with low toxicity and irritation. Good for sore muscles, joint pains, arthritis and hip dysplasia. **Horse** - Gives tone to skeletal muscles and warms any winter chills. Dilates local blood vessels and improves local blood flow to the muscles warming the muscles from inside. Arthritic joints respond well to pepper and helps with pain management when used over a long period of time. Strengthens the nervous system. May antidote Homoeopathics.

Caraway Seed - Good for digestive problems, wind, poor appetite, indigestion and bad breath.

Cardamom - Digestive problems, bad breath. **Horse** - Good for treating digestive problems of a nervous origin. Encourages the flow of saliva and good for loss of appetite. It is warming when the body feels cold and useful for easing coughs and respiratory complaints. Highly antiviral and second only to Eucalyptus in that respect. For stallions you can use it as an aphrodisiac. May irritate some sensitive skins.

Carrot Seed - Valuable oil in the use of skin care, dry flaky skin that is sensitive to allergens and prone to infections. **Horses** - Strengthens the mucous membranes so is good for respiratory conditions. Useful for regenerating the skin after wounds or skin diseases and it antiseptic action will deal with minor infections. Has a toning hormone like action that will encourage conception and assist the infertile mare.

Cedarwood Atlas - Gentle stimulating oil that increases circulation and stimulates the release toxins. Good for the skin and fleas don't like it. **Horse** - Sores that are slow to heal, saddle sores, folliculitis etc. and dry flaky skin, encourage the re-growth of coat and adds shine. Has a tonic effect on the kidneys. Dries out excess phlegm and runny noses and removes excess mucous from the respiratory system when inhaled.

Chamomile German - Powerful skin soothing ant inflammatory. Burns, allergic reaction and all types of skin irritations can be quickly calmed with this oil. The oil has a deep blue color.

Chamomile Roman - Valuable for soothing the central nervous system and relieving cramps spasms and muscle pains. It also has analgesic effects which may be used for wounds. In humans this has traditionally been used for teething. **Horse** - The strong analgesic properties relieve dull muscular aches and stubborn spasms. It can also relieve overworked and inflamed muscles. Can be used as a wash to relieve the pain of inflames wounds. Good for calming difficult and unruly horses. Good for unmanageable mares when they cycle.

Cinnamon Leaf - Use the leaf not the bark as the leaf is gentler. Excellent digestive tonic and good for flatulent dogs and is a powerful anti-microbial.

Citronella - Well known insect repeller.

Clary Sage - Sedates the central nervous system, good for calming blends. **Horse** - Has a strong regenerative power where hair loss is involved. Useful on puffy joints caused by long periods of standing. Any swelling in the kidney area caused by strenuous work or sluggish kidney function. Calms underlying tension and soothes anxiety. Useful for a mare having trouble conceiving or nervous of the stallion. Don't use during pregnancy.

Coriander Seed - A toning balancing and strengthening oil that promotes and supports the digestion. It is also a circulatory stimulant and thus a good addition to blends for sore joints, muscles or arthritis.

Eucalyptus Radiata - A well-known remedy for congestion of the respiratory system. The oil has anti-viral, anti-inflammatory and expectorant effects. Can be a flea repellant. Antidotes Homoeopathic remedies. **Horse** - Eases muscular aches and pains caused by over exertion, relieves rheumatic and nerve pains. The anti-viral action is good for respiratory infections and it also soothes the inflammation and reduces excess mucous. Heals sores prone to pus formation. Can be irritating to sensitive skin.

Frankincense - Used to strengthen a weakened immune system and is a good choice for any blend for a sick or elderly animal that needs a systemic boost. Can be used for skin aliments due to its anti-inflammatory and anti-bacterial qualities. Horse - Eases shortness of breath and helps any respiratory problem. Rejuvenating especially for those recovering from a serious injury, tonic for the aging and can be used as a pick me up. Good for stubborn hard to heal wounds. Has the ability to dispel fear and anxiety. Don't use during pregnancy.

Geranium - Has tonic and strong anti-fungal actions, suitable in the use of prevention and treatment of fungal ear infections. Also can be used in tick repellant formulas. **Horse** - Gentle analgesic, has diuretic properties and a tonic action on the liver and kidneys. Balance hormones and emotions so is good for erratic mood swings.

Ginger - Good for the digestive and circulatory systems. Used for motion sickness, sprains, strains and arthritis. **Horse** - Good for conditions caused by cold and dampness. Stimulates circulation to cold joints and is analgesic relieving arthritic and rheumatic pain, muscle spasms and sprains. Is a appetite stimulant and can relieve travel sickness.
Careful on sensitive skins.

Grapefruit - Used for calming, deodorizing and also repelling insects particularly fleas. Has a tonic effect on skin, hair and tissues. Useful for animals with imbalanced sebum production. **Horse** - Gentle effective lymphatic stimulant that nourishes cells while removing toxins. Tonic to the liver. Careful on sensitive skins.

Helichrysum - Actions - Analgesic, anti-inflammatory, regenerative, good for the skin.

Hyssop Decumbens - Different from the normal hyssop. This one is a antiviral and antibacterial and anti-depressant. The oil is also nontoxic and irritating.

Juniper Berry - Stimulating to the circulatory system and good for use in blends used for arthritis and pain. Helpful for balancing oily skin and for acne, eczema and hair loss. **Horse** - Helps stimulate kidney function and this in turn helps to remove metabolic wastes. Don't use during pregnancy.

Labdunum - This oil is antibacterial and astringent. Used for wounds.

Lavender - Antibacterial, antipruritic (anti-itch), powerful regenerative properties. The oil acts as a sedative on the central nervous system. **Horse** - Is cell regenerating and hastens the healing process. Sedates and soothes any wound or emotion. Helps to dispel gas and eases muscle tightness.

Lemon - Calming, strong antibacterial, deodorizer. **Horse** - Stimulates the body to excrete toxins and wastes via the skin, gently astringent and encourages the movement and release of excess toxins. Supports the liver and kidneys. In the cold season gently addresses runny watery respiratory problems and boosts the immune system. For older horses it can be added to rheumatic blends.

Lemon Grass - Antiviral and has a calming effect. **Horse** - Relieves pain in aching muscles and makes the muscles supple. Careful on sensitive skin and around wounds.

Mandarin Green - Good for calming fear, anxiety or stress. **Horse** - Nourishes the peripheral circulation feeding any extremity that suffers from poor circulation. Helps with muscle spasms.

Marjoram - Calming, spasmolytic, strong antibacterial, bacterial infections, wound care and insect repelling.
Meant to be good for calming over amorous male dogs. **Horse** - Warms cold aching joints, relieves muscle spasms and draws bruising to the surface. Helps with the aches and pain of arthritis and swollen joints in old horses. Can help with travel sickness.

Myrrh - Anti-inflammatory, anti-viral, good for puppy teething, treating irritated or inflamed skin conditions or for adding to immune boosting blends. Good for repelling ticks. **Horse** - Its antiseptic action is useful for deep seated respiratory conditions when inhaled. Can be used in a compress to treat boils, chapped or weeping skin conditions and fungal conditions like ringworm. Has a stimulating toning action on the mares reproductive system. Use only short term and not during pregnancy.

Neroli - Calming, stress reduction, anxiety, used for blend for female dogs in labor to ease pain and stress.

Niaouli - Anti histamine, antibacterial, good for

allergies manifesting on the skin as well as first aid. Use for cleaning and for preventing ear infections in dogs.

Nutmeg - Canine flatulence, reduces gas production and aids in indigestion and nausea. Stimulating to the circulatory system.

Sweet Orange - Calming, deodorizing, flea repellant, may help in excess sebum production of the skin.

Palmarosa - Antibacterial, antiviral. **Horse** - Helpful when the body is over heated, encourages cellular regeneration and aid hydration by encouraging the flow of fluids throughout the body. Good for stiff joints and aching back.

Patchouli - Gentle circulatory stimulant for the skin and coat and also acts as a insect repellant. **Horse** - Tissue regenerator that aids in the healing of wounds, may address old scar tissue if applied regularly. Used for treating sores that contain heat a compress will cool the wound and help heal. Helps the skin regain its elasticity. Has diuretic properties.

Peppermint - Stimulates circulation, analgesic, sprains, strains, arthritis, repels fleas, flies, mossies' , itching, car sickness. **Horse** - Peppermint has a cooling and analgesic action on heated local injuries. Can burn sensitive skins. Antidotes Homoeopathics.

Ravensare - Anti viral and antibacterial. For animals with compromised immune systems or for young dogs that are prone to infections.

Rose - Stabilizing to the central nervous system, has a gentle tonifying effect to the skin good for adding to blends for itchy or irritated skin.

Rosemary - The oil is mucolytic acting as a expectorant and also aids in cell regeneration. May help in promoting and maintaining hair growth. **Horse** - Stimulates both the mental and physical body into action, can relieve pain without sedating.

Rosewood - The oil has antiviral and antibacterial properties and ticks are repelled by the scent of it. Good for skin conditions.

Spearmint - Similar actions to peppermint, repels fleas and other insects stimulates circulation to the area it is used.

Spikenarde - Calming and grounding, rejuvenating and regenerating to the skin, good for dogs with skin problems, has a similar range of action as valerian.

Thyme Linalol - Antibacterial, anti-fungal, good for skin problems and not as harsh as thyme.

Thyme Thujanol - Has all the benefits of the above thyme as well as being a immune system stimulant and live detoxifier. Can be used in the prevention of lymes disease applied immediately after a tick bite.

Valerian - Calming and grounding, good for dogs with separation anxiety or who are fearful of loud noises, storms, fireworks or new situations. Good as a tonic for the nervous system.

Vetiver - Used in blends for calming, circulatory tonic and strengthens the immune system. **Horse** -

Used to treat aches and pains and is a tonic for most body systems. Used for debilitated and distressed horses.

Ylang Ylang - Deeply calming, used in fatigue blends. **Horses** - Commonly used as a aphrodisiac, has an affinity for the adrenal glands.

Notes

Notes

Notes

Notes

Notes

Notes

www.ingramcontent.com/pod-product-compliance
Lightning Source LLC
Chambersburg PA
CBHW071409170526
45165CB00001B/223